But You Look Just Fine

My Journey to Rediscover Joy Amidst Chronic Pain and Invisible Illness

Michele Roys

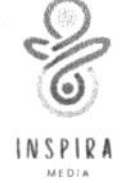

Inspira Media Ltd.

Cover Designed by *Getcovers*

www.micheleroys.com

Limits of Liability and Disclaimer of Warranty:

The authors and/or publisher shall not be liable for your misuse of this material. The contents are strictly for informational and educational purposes only.

Warning—Disclaimer:

The purpose of this book is to educate and entertain. The authors and/or publisher do not guarantee that anyone following these techniques, suggestions, tips, ideas, or strategies will become successful. The author and/or publisher shall have neither liability nor responsibility to anyone with respect to any loss or damage caused, or alleged to be caused, directly or indirectly by the information contained in this book. Further, readers should be aware that Internet websites listed in this work may have changed or disappeared between when this work was written and when it is read.

Printed by an international print-on-demand network

Paperback ISBN: 978-1-0683887-0-5

Hardcover ISBN: 978-1-0683887-2-9

E-book ISBN: 978-1-0683887-1-2

A catalogue record for this book is available from the National Library of Ireland and the Library of Trinity College Dublin.

Disclaimer:

This memoir is based on my personal experiences. While I have made every effort to maintain the accuracy of events, the stories shared here reflect my perspective at the time. Some names and identifying details have been changed to protect the privacy of individuals.

Praise for Memoir

But You Look Just fine

My heart opened completely when I read Michele's beautiful memoir. As someone who knows firsthand what it means to navigate life with an illness, I felt every word of her journey deep in my bones. This isn't just another story about chronic pain—it's a love letter to anyone who's ever felt unseen in their suffering, who's wondered if joy was still possible while living with persistent pain.

Michele's raw honesty about her struggles, her fears, and yes, even her triumphs (because they're there, darling, even on the hardest days) reminds us that healing isn't about reaching some perfect destination. It's about learning to dance with uncertainty, finding moments of light in the darkness, and discovering that our worth isn't tied to our productivity or pain levels.

What I love most about this book is how Michele weaves together practical wisdom with soul-deep truth, showing us that while we can't always control our circumstances, we can choose how we respond to them. Whether you're dealing with chronic pain, supporting someone who is, or simply trying to understand the complex dance between suffering and joy, this book will be your companion, your guide, and your reminder that you are never, ever alone on this journey.

Trust me, this is the kind of book that will make you feel seen, understood, and (most importantly) hopeful. Keep it close to your heart. I know I will.

- **Kris Carr, *New York Times* bestselling author, wellness coach & cancer thriver**

But You Just Look Fine by Michele Roys is an intense and to-the-point exploration of invisible illnesses, shedding light on the often misunderstood world of chronic pain and disease, which I happen to know too well. Michele's world turns upside down as she navigates through disappointing medical treatments, mirroring the frustration and desperation that many face. Her path to healing takes an unexpected turn as she discovers the transformative power of psychotherapy and alternative healing methods.

For me, there are two extremely powerful take-home messages in Michele's story:

First, we sometimes hide behind labels like "Type A" personality, when in truth, we wear this seemingly as a badge of honor. In contrast, we should uncover the insecurities lurking deep below, covering up our true personality.

Secondly, when Michele is confronted after years of suffering with the option of surgery to cure her of all the pain, she takes an unexpected decision that is in full alignment with Eastern philosophy. She exemplifies the expression that the journey is the true objective. She gained so much personal growth and self-acceptance out of the journey, which dwarfs the earlier goal to be just pain-free. It shows her courage and moves me to tears.

This is a must-read for anyone struggling with chronic illness of any sort.

- Dr. PetraFrese, Founder of Peak Mind Academy, Best-selling Author

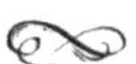

I couldn't put Michele's book, *But You Look Just Fine,* down. As a fellow Autoimmune Disease Warrior, I am all too familiar with the sting of those words—and the silent battles they hide. Michele's story resonated deeply with me, bringing back the confusion, frustration, and overwhelming fear I felt when I first received my diagnosis.

Through her exquisite writing, Michele weaves a powerful narrative of resilience and grace, inviting us into her journey with raw honesty and unwavering courage. Her ability to find strength even when her own body felt foreign is nothing short of inspiring. Page after page, I was awestruck by her tenacity, her hope, and her refusal to give up on herself.

Michele's story isn't just a tale of survival—it's a testament to the human spirit, the healing power of compassion, and the beauty of never losing faith, even in the hardest moments. I'm so honored to know her and incredibly proud of what she's accomplished with this remarkable book.

But You Look Just Fine is more than a memoir; it's a lifeline for anyone navigating the invisible struggles of chronic illness. Michele's words have the power to touch hearts, inspire action, and remind us all that even when we feel unseen, we are never alone.

This book deserves a place on everyone's shelf—and I have no doubt it will become the bestseller it's destined to be.

- Mina GraceWard, Founder of The Graves' Disease Academy, Chef and Author of *There Had to Be Another Way - Things You Didn't Know You Could Do for Graves' Disease* and *The Graves' Disease Chef - How to Master Simple to Gourmet Plant-Based Flavors from Around the World*

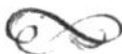

In *But You Look Just Fine*, Michele Roys bravely opens the door to her world, illuminating the often-hidden struggles of living with chronic pain and invisible illness. Her candid narrative resonates deeply, particularly with those of us who—like me—have experienced the relentless push of workaholic tendencies that lead to burnout. As a parent of a son with an autoimmune disease, I understand the critical importance of shining a light on invisible illnesses and educating others about their realities to increase awareness and compassion.

Michele's journey is a powerful reminder that we are not alone in our struggles and that embracing vulnerability can be a path to healing. Her insightful reflections and heartfelt anecdotes provide a roadmap for rediscovering joy amidst adversity. This book is not just a memoir; it's a source of inspiration and hope for anyone who has felt the weight of unacknowledged pain. I highly recommend it to anyone seeking understanding, connection, and the courage to prioritize their well-being. Michele's voice is a beacon of light for those navigating their own difficult journeys.

- Macarena luz Bianchi, Speaker & CEO of Spark Social Press

For anyone who's ever smiled through gritted teeth when hearing "*But You Look Just Fine*", Michele's powerful narrative hits home with stunning precision. As someone who once navigated the maddening maze of an invisible injury while my Type A personality screamed to push forward, I found myself nodding, tearing up, and finally exhaling with relief through these pages. Michele's masterfully captures that surreal disconnect between our external appearance and internal battle – that moment when your body betrays your driven spirit, and the world can't see your daily war.

This isn't just a book; it's a validation, a permission slip to acknowledge the unseen struggles we endure. Michele's insights are like a warm embrace from someone who truly gets it, offering both solace and strategies for those caught in the exhausting dance of looking 'fine' while feeling anything but. Her words will resonate with anyone who's ever felt trapped between their aspirations and their reality, between their capabilities and their constraints.

But You Look Just Fine is the companion I wish I'd had during my darkest days of recovery – a powerful reminder that you're not alone, you're not crazy, and your invisible battle is valid. This book isn't just important; it's essential reading for anyone navigating the complex journey of invisible illness or injury, and for those who love them.

- **Kristin Ericksen, Founder- Break Free Make It Happen**

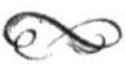

In life, some journeys are marked not by the destinations reached, but by the strength and grace it takes to endure the path. *But You Look Just Fine* by Michele Roys is one such extraordinary journey—a testament to the resilience of the human spirit when faced with the silent battles of chronic pain and invisible illness.

Through this book, Michele opens a door into a world that many endure silently—a world where smiles mask suffering, and the words "But you look just fine" serve as both a compliment and a reminder of isolation. Her courage in sharing the raw truth of her experiences is an act of generosity, offering hope to anyone who has ever felt unseen in their pain.

What makes Michele's story so powerful is not just the adversity she faced, but the wisdom she uncovered along the way. She transforms pain into purpose and shows that even in the darkest valleys, light can break through. Her exploration of holistic therapies, self-compassion, and finding joy amidst life's trials reminds us that healing is not a linear process, but a deeply personal journey toward rediscovering ourselves.

This book is not just for those who live with chronic illness, but for anyone seeking resilience, purpose, and the beauty of finding light in unexpected places. Michele's words will resonate long after you've turned the final page, offering comfort and inspiration to those who need it most.

Michele's memoir is an invitation to live with courage, to embrace our stories, and to find joy in the moments that define us—not despite our struggles, but because of them. Let her journey inspire yours.

With Gratitude,

- Lia Valencia Key, Founder of VALENCIA KEY

Michele Roys' book, *But You Look Just Fine*, takes us on a journey deep into what it's like to look good on the outside and yet be sick and feel broken. She dives into the heart of bringing us back to joy and true living regardless of the diagnosis. This is a must read to discover the power of self-love and possibility and to be able to share itso others can understand.

- Carol Register, SINC Certified Master Neurocoach™

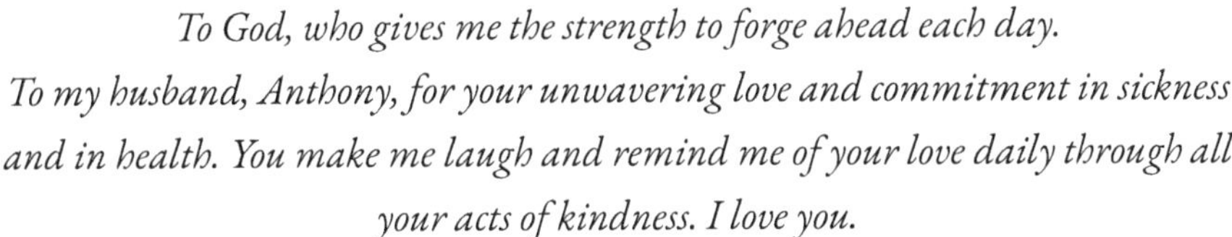

To God, who gives me the strength to forge ahead each day.

To my husband, Anthony, for your unwavering love and commitment in sickness and in health. You make me laugh and remind me of your love daily through all your acts of kindness. I love you.

To Collin and Ryan, my dear sons, for your love, continued encouragement, and belief in me. I love you, and I am so proud of you both.

Contents

Introduction

Dear Reader,

Thank you for choosing to open this book and walk with me through my journey. It means so much to me, yet this story isn't just about me—it's about you, too. *But You Look Just Fine* is for anyone who has ever felt unseen or misunderstood in their pain, anyone who has struggled to hold onto hope. I wrote these words to be a companion for you, a reminder that you don't have to face this alone.

This book began as a private journal, a space where I could pour out my frustration and confusion over what was happening to me. Each day, I faced constant pain. I visited countless doctors, underwent seemingly endless exams, and dealt with a cycle of waiting for answers that never seemed to come. I felt isolated, overwhelmed, and sometimes questioned if I could keep going.

The weight of it all was suffocating, and there were moments when it felt like too much to bear. But in one of those darkest moments, I felt a sense of calm—like a quiet assurance from God that He would make a way if I could trust Him and allow the deeper work to unfold within me.

Gradually, my journaling evolved into something more—a purpose. I began writing for someone I imagined, someone like me, who might also be feeling lost, tired, and in need of hope. I wanted this book to serve as a roadmap, a companion for anyone navigating a similar path who might need a reminder that healing and joy are still possible. This single focus became my motivation, and over the past three years, I wrote with the hope and prayer that these words would be a source of comfort and encouragement for others who are searching for answers and strength.

This book is written in five parts, each reflecting a stage in my journey with chronic pain—a journey that mirrored the stages of grief. I walked through denial, anger, bargaining, and finally arrived at acceptance and the rediscovery of joy. Alongside my story of pain, I share how I worked through childhood trauma, reconnected with the essence of who I am, and learned to live in a new way.

As you read, I hope you'll connect with my story and recognize the strength within yourself. These words were written for you. When I finally began to let go of control and opened my heart to love, compassion, and gentleness, my journey transformed. The path became less about surviving and more about truly living, with joy becoming possible once again.

Above all, my hope is that this book will encourage you not to give up. May it bring awareness to the unseen challenges of invisible illness, and may it inspire those living with chronic pain to rediscover joy. You are worthy. You are never alone. I believe in you, and I am honoured to be here with you.

With love and light,

Michele Roys

Part 1: The Breakdown

"Perfectionism is a self destructive and addictive belief system that fuels this primary thought: If I look perfect, and do everything perfectly, I can avoid or minimize the painful feelings of shame, judgment, and blame."
– **Brené Brown,** *The Gifts of Imperfection*

Chapter 1

Warning Signs

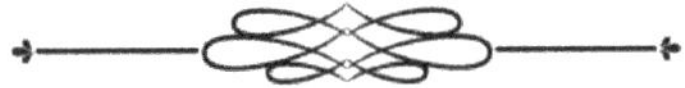

"Mom, we're having panettone for breakfast, and there's barely any left for you. Come quick!"

Collin's voice drifts up the stairs, and my heart leaps at the mention of panettone. That sweet Italian bread, the taste of Christmases at my grandmother's, the comfort of childhood wrapped in a paper wrapping. I'm out of bed in seconds, rushing down our curved staircase in my fluffy slippers, mind already tasting that cherished treat—

Then my world tilts.

My left leg skids from under me. My right foot catches behind, and I scramble for the banister as I slide down seven steps. The thunderous thump of my landing brings my husband and boys running from the kitchen. They find me curled at the base of the stairs, clutching my right foot, mind struggling to process what just happened.

Now, less than two months later, the searing pain that shoots up from my toes to my spine threatens to crumble me, but I can't stop. I have to get to work.

The ever-present voice in my head urges me to push through the agony. *Come on, Michele! Mind over matter. You can't let anyone think you're lazy or incapable.*

I'm driving from Limerick to Wicklow on a frigid January morning, the commute stretching two and a half hours ahead of me. Only fifteen minutes in, my right foot is screaming with every press of the accelerator. Tony Robbins drones through the speakers, but his motivational words fade beneath the rhythm of my mantras: "All things are possible" and "When I am weak, then I am strong."

My husband's worried face flashes in my mind. This morning, he'd stood in our kitchen, coffee cup frozen halfway to his lips as he watched me prepare to leave. "You're not ready," he'd said simply. "The doctor said eight weeks minimum." But I'd smiled, kissed his cheek, and promised I'd be fine. I couldn't tell him how my recent promotion after only three months at work felt like a tightrope—one wrong move and I'd fall into the abyss of being seen as incapable, unreliable.

The bulky protective boot sits hidden behind my seat, a reminder of my weakness. At work, where I serve as HR Generalist—doing the job of an HR manager but without the title—I'll have to wear it. But for now, I press my broken toe against the pedal, each movement sending shockwaves of pain up my leg.

Your friends are telling you to slow down, Michele. Your husband, too, not to mention your doctors and physiotherapist.

Don't they understand I can't stop? If I do, I might crumble. I've defined myself as a driven, career-oriented woman for years now. And so, I forge on. *If you don't listen to the pain, you won't feel it,* I reason with myself, even as my sciatic nerve screams in protest.

My boys' faces swim before my eyes—Ryan's quiet concern, Collin's lingering guilt over the panettone call that sent me tumbling. But I push those thoughts away. I can't let pain stop me. I can't let my family's worry hold me back. I have to prove I'm strong enough, capable enough, worthy of this promotion.

And so I drive on, one excruciating mile at a time, pretending all is well, while my body keeps its own brutal score.

The memory of that Sunday in the Accident & Emergency unit floods back as I grip the steering wheel tighter. I'd insisted on driving myself there, waving away the concerned father at Collin's rugby practice who'd offered help. "I'll be fine," I'd said, forcing a smile, while Collin watched me struggle with crutches on the muddy field. Always fine. Always capable. Always strong.

The senior nurse's words echo in my head: "You're very lucky not to have done more damage in the fall. Take the time your body is asking for now, and you'll be much better in the long run." But I'd dismissed her wisdom just as I'd dismissed the concerned father, my husband's worry, my children's fear. The X-ray had shown a clean break above the joint in my big toe, but I saw something different in those stark white images—I saw weakness, vulnerability, a threat to everything I'd worked so hard to build.

A slow car in front of me forces me to brake, and I bite back a cry. The morning traffic crawls around me, each stop and start a fresh torture. But I keep my face composed, my lipstick perfect, my clothes professional. No one looking through my car window would guess that each press of the pedal sends lightning bolts of pain through my body. No one would know that beneath my polished exterior, I'm waging a war between my body's demands and a relentless drive to prove myself.

My boss's words replay in my mind: "You can work from home. Take the time you need." His offer had been generous, understanding. But all I'd heard was pity, a threat to my carefully constructed image of competence. I'd rather drive two and a half hours in agony than let anyone think I couldn't handle my responsibilities.

God is my rescue and my strength, I remind myself as I continue down the main highway. But even as I pray these words, a small voice whispers: *Who are you really trying to prove yourself to? And at what cost?*

I silence that voice just as I silence the pain. There's work to be done, meetings to attend, a new position to justify. I reach to adjust the rear-view mirror and catch a glimpse of my face—composed, determined, hiding the storm beneath. Just as I've hidden the protective boot, just as I've hidden my medical certificate recommending six to eight weeks of rest, just as I've hidden every grimace and tear of pain these past two months.

The highway stretches ahead, a ribbon of asphalt leading to another day of pretending, pushing, proving. The sun rises over the Irish countryside, painting the sky in shades of pink and gold, but I barely notice its beauty. All I can focus on is maintaining this careful balance between agony and ambition, between family and career, between the person I think I need to be and the person my body is begging me to become.

Each mile marker that passes is another small victory, another proof that I'm winning this battle against weakness. The familiar exit signs tick by: Portlaoise, Kildare, Naas. My toe throbs in time with my heartbeat, but I focus on my breathing, on my plans for the day ahead, on anything but the growing chorus of pain in my body.

The medical certificate sits in my bedside drawer at home, its recommendation for six to eight weeks of rest a mockery of everything I believe about myself. Six weeks of rest might heal a broken toe, but what would it do to my reputation? To my chances of advancement? To my very identity?

I think of my grandmother, how she would lay out the panettone each Christmas, her hands moving with careful grace even as arthritis twisted her fingers. "Listen to your body, pequena," she would say. "It speaks wisdom." But I've spent years training myself not to listen, to push through, to prove myself in a world that seems to demand ever more.

The morning sun finally breaks through the clouds as I approach Wicklow, bathing the office buildings in golden light. I park in my usual spot, carefully hidden from the main entrance where colleagues might see me struggling with the crutches. I'll wait until the morning rush has passed before I make my way inside. Then I'll exchange my flat shoe for the protective boot, plaster on a smile, and begin another day of careful pretence.

You're doing the right thing, I tell myself as I sit in the car, gathering strength for the performance ahead. *You're being responsible. Professional. Strong.*

But as I reach for my bag, a spasm of pain shoots from my toe up through my leg, and for just a moment, my carefully constructed facade cracks. A single tear escapes before I can catch it, dropping onto my crisp white blouse. I quickly dab it away, reapply my lipstick, check my reflection one final time.

The woman in the mirror looks perfect, composed, ready to take on the world. Only I know the cost of maintaining this image. Only I can feel the warning signals my body is sending, growing louder with each passing day. But I ignore them all, just as I've always done.

After all, I remind myself as I reach for the door handle, what's one more broken piece when you're fighting to keep everything from falling apart?

Chapter 2

Tipping Point

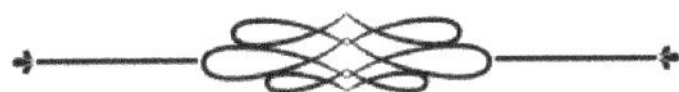

"I'm still standing," I tell my doctor, trying to hold back tears. They stream down my face anyway. My body shivers with cold while a high temperature has left me feeling like a melting snowman. My headache is unbearable, my chest hurts, and I'm exhausted.

"You have a terrible chest infection and sinusitis, and it won't get better without rest," he says, looking at me with concern. After ten years as my doctor, he knows me well enough to anticipate my response.

"I can work from bed. That's rest, right?" The words come out hoarse, but I manage a smile. Even as I speak, my mind races through deadlines, meetings, and responsibilities waiting for me. *Just power through*, I tell myself. *Mind over matter*.

But my body has other plans. The past two months of 2018 have finally caught up with me, demanding payment for all the times I've pushed aside its warnings. My throat constricts as I think about how I got here, about all the storms—both literal and metaphorical—I've weathered recently.

Three weeks earlier, the "Beast from the East" had turned Ireland into a winter wonderland—beautiful from behind a window, hazardous from behind a wheel. Making my weekly 250-kilometer commute from Dublin to Limerick, I found myself facing conditions I'd never encountered in my years of driving. In Brazil, where I grew up, snow existed only in movies and postcards. Now it was all too real, transforming familiar roads into treacherous paths.

I gripped the steering wheel until my knuckles turned white, my car skidding slightly as I eased onto the corner road. "Gears, not brakes," I muttered to myself, remembering advice I'd read online. Fresh snow pelted the windshield as I inched down the highway, prayers tumbling from my lips in a mixture of Portuguese and English.

"You've got this," I whispered to myself, the words becoming a rhythm matching my windshield wipers. "Just like everything else, you've got this." The mantra helped steady my nerves as cars whizzed past, their drivers seemingly oblivious to the dangerous conditions. Each time one passed, my heart jumped into my throat, but I kept going. I had to—my job in HR didn't stop for snow, and neither could I.

That drive should have been my warning sign, my body's first attempt to tell me to slow down. But I didn't listen. I couldn't. Not when my world turned upside down just days later.

It was Saturday, and we'd taken the boys to the University of Limerick grounds for sledding. While they played in the snow, I paced near the hill, phone pressed to my ear, coordinating with another manager about staffing shortages. I'd been working remotely since the storm hit, trying to ensure essential services continued despite the weather.

"Just one more run," I'd called out to the boys, gesturing toward the café where hot chocolates awaited. They climbed onto their makeshift sled together, bundled in winter jackets and gloves, their cheeks red from cold and excitement.

Then it happened—a moment that seemed to unfold in slow motion. I was mid-sentence about staff coverage when I saw their sled veer off course. The sickening crack as it hit the fence post. Collin's arm connecting with the concrete fence top. My twelve-year-old's scream cut through the winter air, and I watched the colour drain from his face even before I reached him.

"I'll call you back," I managed to say into the phone before dropping it into my pocket. Through layers of winter clothing, we couldn't see the extent of the injury, but Collin's face and the way he cradled his arm told us enough. We carefully helped him inside the café, and only when we managed to ease off his jacket did we see the true damage—his arm bent at an impossible angle.

My husband, ever practical, found a wooden spoon in the café and created a makeshift splint while I tried to keep Collin calm. Though the skin hadn't broken, his wrist pointed one way, his arm another. My younger son sat, crying from his own collision with the fence. Though his injuries weren't immediately visible, the shock had left him in tears. Later, we would discover the severe bruising on his leg and ankle, but in that moment, all I could do was try to stay calm for both my boys. Even as I rushed to the hospital, emails pinged on my phone—urgent messages about staff shortages at work, nurses unable to reach work due to weather conditions.

In the paediatric ward, harsh fluorescent lights cast everything in an unnatural glow. The steady beep of monitors created a backdrop to my frantically typed emails and whispered phone calls. Four screws and a metal plate now held my son's bones together. Collin handled it with remarkable bravery, even managing weak jokes about being part cyborg now.

The room held four other children and their mothers. I felt their eyes on me every time my phone rang, their disapproval heavy in the air as I coordinated with local guards to transport essential staff to work. Between calls to arrange replacement nurses and updating work schedules, I'd carry Collin his tablet and headphones, trying to make up for my divided attention with small gestures.

"You earned some technology time," I'd say, adjusting his pillows before ducking into the hallway for another urgent call. In quiet moments, guilt gnawed at me—guilt for not being fully present for my son, guilt for not being at work, guilt for every task left undone.

Every email I answered, every staffing gap I filled, meant another vulnerable child with severe disabilities would receive the care they desperately needed. These children depended on consistent care and familiar faces. I couldn't let them down, even as my own body protested. The hospital chair transformed into my office, its hard plastic edges digging into my back as I balanced my laptop. Night fell, and the ward's sounds changed. My senses adjusted to the shuffle of nurses' shoes, the soft whimpers of pain, the hum of machines. Sleep came in snatches, interrupted by work emergencies and nurses checking Collin's vitals.

The next morning brought my own orthopaedic consultation in the same hospital. Between managing my injury and Collin's recovery, work piled up like the snow outside. But I kept going. I had to. There was no other choice.

Now, sitting in my doctor's office weeks later, my body stages its rebellion. Each breath feels like inhaling glass, and the fever burns through my pretences of invincibility. The infection that's taken root in my chest seems to mock all my carefully constructed illusions of control.

"Please," my doctor says, his voice gentler now, "you need to actually rest this time. Not work-from-bed rest. Real rest."

I nod, already planning how to manage my workload from home. He hands me a prescription, his expression a mixture of concern and resignation. He's seen this determination in me before, this refusal to yield.

The antibiotics rattle in their package as I make my way home, each step a battle against exhaustion. But even as fever burns through me, I open my laptop. Emails need answering. Reports need reviewing. The world won't stop spinning just because I'm sick.

"I am strong," I whisper through another coughing fit, the words raspy and raw. "I am capable. I can do this."

The mantra sounds as tired as I feel, but I keep typing anyway. The screen blurs before my eyes, and my head pounds with each keystroke. But I'm still standing—or at least, sitting upright enough to work. In my mind, that counts as rest. Tomorrow will be better. It has to be. Because stopping isn't an option I'm willing to consider. Not yet. Not ever.

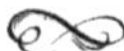

It is August of 2018, and I've just come back from a three-week vacation with family and friends in the USA and Canada. We had a great time, but—as is often the case with vacations—it wasn't exactly restful. Now, back in Ireland, it's the hottest summer we've had in years. Farmers are complaining about the drought and the heat, yet here I am with a condition usually reserved for winter flu.

I've been hit with a chest infection I can't seem to shake. The doctor is concerned I might have pneumonia and orders an X-ray. My chest hurts, I can't stop coughing, and it's painful to swallow, but I'm in the middle of revising company policies due to go before the board of directors next week. Why is my body fighting me when it knows I can't take a break?

I sit in a dark room with closed curtains at two in the afternoon. My sore eyes make it painful to look at my computer screen, but I continue to revise the documents. My phone rings, jolting me from my work. Grateful for the opportunity to rest my eyes for a few moments, I greet my colleague and try to keep up with the conversation. But I can't stop coughing.

"Michele, shouldn't you be resting? You don't sound too good." I brush off his concern, telling him I can work on the policy revisions from bed. As soon as I end the call, I'm left alone with my thoughts again. They grow increasingly dark.

Tears come, burning my tired eyes. I let them flow. Why is my body making it so hard for me to keep going? All I want to do is remain productive and busy, to prove myself. When others tell me I don't sound well or look well, I feel frustration rising within me. *Thanks for stating the obvious.*

It feels like pieces of me are exposed when I leave work undone. If I stop or even slow down, it will show that I'm not good enough. Not strong enough. Like Dory in the Disney cartoon, I have to just keep swimming.

As long as I refuse to acknowledge the discomfort, the difficulty, the pain, I can convince myself that maybe it will just go away. I swipe the tears from my face. No time for those, either. I need to be strong in my mind in order to keep my body going. But the frustration refuses to leave.

Why can't I push through this like I push through everything else?

Why is my body failing me when I need it the most?

Why can't I be stronger?

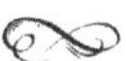

Showing myself as strong and capable has always been important to me. My parents were traveling missionaries, constantly on the go, so we moved to a different part of Brazil every six months or so. As the second oldest of six siblings, I felt a sense of responsibility toward my younger siblings. I also felt the pressure to be perfect. With my parents frequently away, other people often took care of us. I learned quickly that to avoid punishment, I had to be the good girl, always obedient, always striving to meet expectations or risk a spanking.

In my desire to be accepted, I learned to follow orders without question. I was the dependable one, the child who never stepped out of line, hoping my compliance would earn the love and approval I desperately craved. I felt a constant need to excel, to be the best at everything, driven by an inner voice that whispered, *You're not enough.*

Beneath this all was a deep-seated fear of God. I strove to be good not just for my parents and caregivers, but also for Him, hoping to earn His favour and love. The insecurity of moving so often, never having a stable home, made me cling even harder to this desire to be perfect.

One day when I was four years old, I went to São Paulo with my mom. I held her hand as we walked along a path lined with vibrant hibiscus flowers. I wore a white dress with black polka-dots, my white socks pulled up neatly from shiny black shoes. The feel of my mom's hand in mine was reassuring, for the moment; she spent so much time away from home in her mission work. Was she going to leave again?

We passed green bushes and towering palm trees. My mom asked me to wait on a bench and walked away. Sitting there by myself, I felt small and a little anxious, knowing that I needed to be on my best behaviour. The world around me was vast and unpredictable, yet I knew my role: to be quiet and obedient.

Time dragged on, but eventually my mom returned with a flower tucked into her hair and a big smile on her face. Beside her was a man with blond, curly hair, light eyes, and a warm smile.

"Michele, this is your new father," she said, her smile widening.

I looked up at him, extending my hand with a mix of curiosity and unease. *My new dad.* The thought raced through my mind. *Does this mean I can also be replaced?*

My Type A personality began to take shape here, in this moment of silent struggle. It was built upon through many darker moments that followed. Every achievement became a brick in the wall I constructed around my insecurities. I focused on school, activities, and responsibilities, believing that if I could be perfect, I would finally feel worthy. Yet, no matter how hard I tried, the feeling of inadequacy always lingered, pushing me to strive even harder.

I carried this drive into adulthood as a relentless force that directed my path. A double-edged sword, it gave me the strength to push through challenges but also carved deep scars into my sense of self-worth. The need to prove myself was a constant companion, urging me forward even when I was weary from the journey.

And it had been quite the journey so far.

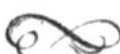

My husband and I moved from London to Ireland in late 2008, when Collin was a toddler and I was nearly eight months pregnant with Ryan. We were basically starting over. The pregnancy tested my limits—carrying a large baby on my petite frame, fighting relentless back pain and sciatica, battling nausea that lingered far beyond the first trimester. Yet even then, I couldn't stay still. That first Christmas, I choreographed children's holiday shows and organized carolling performances for nursing homes—everything perfectly orchestrated, down to the synchronized hand motions.

The real challenge came when I started looking for work in Limerick. Being home with my boys while my husband worked as a sole trader made me restless, but I soon discovered a harsh reality: my decade of managerial experience across three continents meant nothing here. My qualifications weren't recognized. I would have to start from scratch.

Rather than admit defeat, I carved my own path. It started small—weekly visits to a local nursing home with Collin and baby Ryan. The residents' faces lit up at the sight of children, and soon one nursing home became seven. Hope in Motion grew from this seed: a team of mothers and children performing during holidays, bringing joy to the elderly. When the number of handmade cards we needed for residents grew too large for our small group, I enlisted help from my son's school, turning it into a community effort.

But it wasn't enough. That familiar voice whispered: *You're not enough.* In 2012, I enrolled in university fulltime, pursuing a business degree. The juggling act intensified—running Hope in Motion, raising two boys, supporting my husband, and now tackling business math in the learning centre until the numbers finally made sense. I launched "Adopt a Grandfriend," connecting university volunteers with nursing home residents. I co-founded Enactus UL, expanding our impact to include recording elderly residents' life stories and supporting children's initiatives in Thailand. I even joined a local choir, because why not add one more thing to the mix?

When the first Outstanding Scholar Award invitation arrived in the mail, I stared at it in disbelief. There had to be a mistake. I checked the envelope twice, convinced it was meant for someone else. Top of the class? Me? I'd spent countless nights at the kitchen table after the boys were in bed, textbooks spread out, fighting to understand complex business concepts. I'd practically lived in the math learning centre, asking questions until my professors probably grew tired of my voice. Each high mark felt like a happy accident, a result of being older than my classmates, or maybe the professors just took pity on the mature student with two kids.

The next year, another invitation came. I told myself it was a fluke—maybe fewer students that year, maybe the courses were easier. By the third award, I still couldn't shake the feeling of being an impostor. Even as I walked across the stage to accept each award, even as I saw my name at the top of class lists, that childhood voice whispered: *They'll find out you're not really that smart. You just work harder than everyone else.*

Every President's Volunteer Award felt somehow unearned, despite the countless hours invested. I graduated with a first-class honour's degree, but instead of satisfaction, I felt the pressure to push harder, reach further, prove more.

My patient husband watched as I accepted a demanding position after graduation, the culmination of my placement year's networking. Five years of academic excellence, multiple awards, and extensive community impact weren't enough to quiet that childhood voice questioning my worth. And so I pushed on, stretched further, reached higher—until my body finally staged its rebellion.

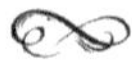

It is early September of 2018, and I arrive at a work conference two minutes behind schedule. My heart races as I rush down the long corridor towards the conference room. But first, a quick bathroom stop.

I thrust the door open in a hurry, trapping my pinkie finger between the door handle and the unforgiving black marble wall. Searing pain jolts through me so intensely that my body starts to tremble. But there's no time to nurse this injury; I'm already running late. I squeeze my pinkie to ease the pain as I make my way to the conference room.

I manage to secure some ice cubes and a towel from a helpful waiter, but as I sit and listen to the keynote speaker, I realize I'm in a bad position. This is a networking event; I can't afford not to shake hands. I will have to brush off the inconvenience of a possibly fractured pinkie and pretend all is well.

After the keynote ends, I stand and make my way around the room, meeting new people. Each time I shake someone's hand, pain shoots up my arm like an electric shock. I try to hide it, to breathe slowly and stay composed.

The room presses in around me, with the chattering of voices and the clack of high heels on hard floors. The tables are set with white cloth, lending an air of grandeur to the event, but all I can focus on is the throbbing ache in my pinkie. Why, of all days, did I have to get injured today?

I refuse to let the pain show. If I tell anyone I hurt myself, it might reflect poorly on me. So, I grit my teeth and continue around the room, enduring 50 handshakes or more during the course of the day. Some firm and unyielding, others weak and limp. *Mind over matter*, I tell myself.

At one point, I introduce myself to a woman with soft makeup, blonde hair, and a scattering of freckles. As she extends her hand, I force a smile and try to maintain my composure. But the pain is too much. A tear escapes the corner of my eye. I cut our conversation short and grab a glass of cold water, dipping my pinkie in the cup to ease the throbbing. Thankfully, no one seems to notice.

By the time I stumble through the door of my rented room near Dublin, tears stream down my face—pent-up agony from a day filled with torturous handshakes. I wish my husband was here to comfort me and tell me it's going to be all right, but he's home in Limerick with our boys. Home never felt so far away.

Chapter 3

Tug of War

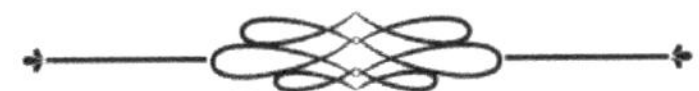

As I arrive at the local rugby club's Family Day Out on a late September day in 2018, I am preoccupied, thinking about work and an upcoming breakfast meeting with my CEO. But I have promised myself to be present in my sons' activities whenever I can, and my husband and both boys are so excited about this event. I force myself to slow down and take a deep breath.

The sweet-and-sour tang of BBQ permeates the air, and the warmth of the sun envelops us. Rugby pitches have been converted into a playground for the kids while surrounding stalls offer hot dogs, BBQ, popcorn, and all sorts of games.

Collin dashes towards the festivities, and Ryan heads after him. It's delightful to see the boys laughing and playing with other kids. It's been far too long since I allowed myself a day to just enjoy my family like this. I watch young kids running up and down to get into line for the bouncy castles while older boys show off their rugby skills, kicking the ball between posts.

I spot my friend Mindy across the field, her black hair catching the sunlight as she waves me over. As I approach, she flashes me a warm smile.

"Hi, Mindy! How's it going?" I ask, trying to shake off the lingering thoughts of work.

"Oh, you know, the usual chaos," she laughs, rolling her eyes. "Chasing after the kids, keeping up with their schedules. How about you? Surviving the weekly commute to Dublin?"

I chuckle. "Barely. I have a big meeting tomorrow, but I couldn't miss today. The boys would never forgive me."

Mindy nods. "I hear you. The twins have been talking about this Family Day for weeks. They practically dragged me out of the house this morning."

We both glance over at our kids. Collin is showing off his rugby skills while Ryan has disappeared into one of the bounce castles. I hear his laughter among the laughter and shouts of other children.

A lady with a bright green shirt, signifying her as one of the volunteers, approaches Mindy and me. "Hey, we're looking for moms to join in a game of tug of war."

I shake my head.

"You should come," Mindy says. She jogs over to join the group of moms. I watch as more mothers are drawn to the big rope that lies on the grass just a few feet from me.

One lady calls out to me. "Your friend has already been roped in. No pun intended!" I laugh and decline, cradling a cup of warm tea.

"We're missing one person on this side," Mindy urges. "Come on!"

I reluctantly agree. How hard can it be? It is all moms like me, on both sides. Husbands and kids are on the sidelines, watching and cheering us on.

I set down my cup of tea and pick up the rope. My mind zeros in on the competition. As soon as the 'go' signal is given, I feel a surge of energy flowing through my veins. I start to pull as hard as I can, determined to win. My hands grip the rope, but as I tug with all my might, I feel a burst of pain in my back. I bite my bottom lip. It feels if my spine is literally being pulled apart.

I release my grip a bit, but as I do, I feel the tension on the rope ease. My whole team is letting go!

I start to shout above the cheers, "Heave, heave, come on, heave!" I take a firmer hold of the rope and keep pulling, digging my heels into the soft ground to get better momentum, screaming "Heave!" all the while. The mothers behind and in front keep pulling.

Determined to help our team make some headway, I ignore the back pain by focusing on the two women in front of me. Inch by inch, we manage to drag the opposing team closer to our side. Victory is within our grasp. But then, a rugby player joins the other side, threatening to turn the tables on us.

I dig my feet deeper into the ground, refusing to let the other team gain ground. My back screams in agony, but I push through.

"Come on, we can do this!" I shout, willing my teammates to push harder. Just when I think I can't take it anymore, we make one last concerted pull, and the other team concedes defeat.

I feel a rush of elation, my heart pounding with excitement. But my victory has come at a price. As I release the rope and try to straighten, my lower back throbs with pain. It feels as though my spine can hardly support the weight of my upper back and shoulders.

I walk toward my friend slowly, compensating for the pain by holding myself in a weird position.

"Are you okay?" Mindy asks.

"I think I hurt my back." I try to smile so as not to alarm her or anyone else. I put both hands on my lower back to give it support.

"I can go find some ice for you. Just wait here." My friend disappears into the crowd. I can barely move, so I stand where she left me, watching people come and go. I hear kids laughing and enjoying themselves on the bouncing castles, about three metres from where I stand. I try to focus on their joy, but the pain is growing worse by the minute.

Finally, Mindy arrives with a paramedic eating a hotdog and holding a soda. "Do you mind following me to the ambulance?" he asks. "I can see what we have there to help you."

I nod and walk slowly behind him, mortified that others can see me walking towards the ambulance. Forget the pain that's making it difficult to move, I'm struggling more with the feeling of being judged.

I catch a glimpse of my husband, Anthony, talking to another friend. Although I hope to pass by without him noticing me, he looks over and spots me.

"Where are you going? Are you okay?" he asks.

"I hurt my back a little," I say, trying to make light of the pain. "I'm just getting some ice for it."

He nods and turns back to his friend, continuing their conversation. Clearly, I am doing well at concealing how bad I actually feel.

Every step is a struggle. I focus on the yellow and green ambulance parked not too far away. It seems like an eternity before I reach it. The driver, a training doctor, and the paramedic who offered me help earlier all wait for me by the ambulance.

"So, what happened?" the main paramedic asks.

I tell him the story. He laughs. Probably thinks I'm crazy.

"Why didn't you let go of the rope when you first felt the pain?" he asks.

"We would have lost," I reply.

The paramedic raises an eyebrow, then looks me over. "An ice pack isn't going to help you now. Look at how you're standing; your axis is out of alignment, and you're overcompensating. I think you're in more pain than you're letting us know."

He's right. I'm in a public space surrounded by friends, children, and strangers. I can't allow the pain to take over now.

I try to conceal my frustration. "I need to drive to Dublin tonight for work. Can you give me a painkiller or two? I can have a good night's rest and hopefully be better tomorrow."

"Are you for real?" he asks. "The worst thing you can do is drive that many hours when you've just hurt your back. From the looks of it, the injury is a lot worse than you are letting on!"

I explain how important it is for me to be at work and ask again if there is anything he can do to help the pain go away. He shakes his head. "We need to see what's going on first. Then we can try to help you get back home tonight."

I finally agree, and he extends his hands to guide me up the ambulance ramp. Every step is agonising, as if my body is made of lead and I am dragging it up inch by inch. I grip his hand tightly, trying to use it as an anchor to keep from falling apart. The other paramedic notices my struggle and offers his arm for support.

Mindy, who remained with me all the while, rushes off to find Anthony.

"Can you lift your arms?" the paramedic asks me. Even that small movement feels like an insurmountable task. As he helps me sit down, a surge of pain explodes through me. I let out a sharp cry and try to calm myself with a series of deep breaths.

"I can't even sit down," I whimper. *Why did I play that stupid game?* I grit my teeth, determined not to let the pain consume me.

When Mindy returns with Anthony, I can see the worry on their faces.

The paramedic motions for me to lie down, and I try to comply; it proves to be a near-impossible task. He supports me with both arms and helps me lie down on the stretcher. I wince as the movement sends a fresh wave of pain coursing through my body. I bite my lip, trying to hold back tears as they close the back doors of the ambulance.

The paramedic hands me some medication to ease my pain, and I gratefully accept. I decline the "green whistle," an inhaled medication used to treat severe pain, not wanting to lose control completely. He explains that I need to go to the hospital. I can't sit. I can't stand. I have no option but to agree.

The paramedic steps outside and a moment later, my husband pops his face inside the small space. "You'll be okay. I will come to the hospital after I sort out the kids."

I nod, still trying to portray strength and keep a sense of control. As we set off towards the hospital, I groan at every bump in the road. *Is this really happening?* The afternoon started off with such promise, but then it all fell apart. My body betrayed me *again*, and now I'm being carted off to the hospital in an ambulance!

The pain is relentless, shooting up my back and down my legs. I'm frustrated with myself for not being able to handle this injury like a boss. The thought of being a burden to Anthony and the boys is overwhelming. I'm supposed to be the mother, the caregiver, not the patient.

My mind races ahead to all the things I need to do. Meetings, deadlines, and so many responsibilities. Yet my life has been turned upside down by a silly game of tug-of-war.

The paramedic sitting next to me tries to make small talk, but my mind is too consumed to engage in conversation. I don't want to hear about the ambulance's terrible suspension or the paramedic's plans for the evening. All I want is to be pain-free and back to my normal routine.

When we arrive at the hospital, the doors of the ambulance open. "This is going to be bumpy," the paramedic warns. As they jostle the trolley, wheeling me into the hospital, I can't help but let out a few moans. The paramedic offers me the green whistle again, but I refuse it.

The trainee doctor and paramedic ask to speak with the triage nurse as I'm taken through the back entrance of the Accident & Emergency (A&E) department for the regional hospital. I can feel my bladder filling up quickly.

"Do you think there's any chance I can go to the bathroom?" I ask the ambulance driver, who is standing near me.

"If you can stand up, we can get the healthcare assistant to go with you," he responds.

"I can go to the bathroom on my own," I protest, annoyed at the suggestion that I need help from a healthcare assistant (HCA).

The triage nurse arrives, and the paramedic informs her that I've refused the green whistle and only took Nurofen and paracetamol about an hour ago.

"She's a tough one." He looks at me. "You sure you don't want the green whistle?"

"I just need to go to the bathroom," I say. "I was drinking tea, and I think the fullness of my bladder is putting extra pressure on my lower back. It's getting very uncomfortable." An understatement.

"We need to change you to a hospital trolley anyway, so we can see if you're able to stand up. If so, you can go to the bathroom. Otherwise, we'll call the HCA to provide another way," he explains.

"What other way?" I ask. The idea of needing help to pee makes me cringe inwardly.

"They can assist you while you're lying down," he responds.

"No way!" I am appalled at the thought of not being able to use the bathroom on my own. "Just give me a hand to lift myself up."

But the slightest movement sends pain shooting all over my body. *There's no way I'm going to get up*, I realise, but I can't bring myself to accept it. I need to go to the bathroom on my own two feet! *I can do this. Come on, body, please work with me! Please God, help me get up ...*

As I try to lift myself to a sitting position, the pain takes over, and I scream out. I grab the paramedic's hands and shoulder, trying to ease the pain by holding on for dear life.

I feel tears start to flow, overwhelmed by the struggle to accept my inability to move.

A hospital trolley with metal frames is wheeled toward me. A healthcare assistant places a white sheet on it. The trolley I am lying on is narrow, and I know I need to be shifted to the other trolley, but how? I cannot move without intense, shooting pain.

Medical professionals, including a paramedic, a trainee doctor, the triage nurse, and a healthcare assistant, surround me, waiting for my signal that I'm ready to be moved.

"Okay, let's do this again, together." The paramedic offers his right hand and supports my neck and upper back with his left hand. I try to lift myself into a sitting position, but the pain takes over, shooting up and down my spine. Grabbing onto the paramedic again, I try to ease the pain by allowing him to lift me. I scream, the pain unbearable. My bladder feels like it is about to explode.

The paramedic pulls a green whistle from his red bag and looks into my eyes. "You need this. Just breathe in deeply. We need to move you to the other trolley." I am now awkwardly positioned half on the original bed and half cradled in his arms while tears stream down my face.

I inhale the magic green whistle, hoping for some relief, while the medical professionals try to shift me to the other trolley. Each move brings excruciating pain, but I try to focus on the whistle and not let the pain take over.

They manage to transfer me to the hospital trolley, and I quietly thank them for their help. The triage nurse explains that two healthcare assistants will assist me in relieving myself, but it will have to be in the bed. "I'm sorry," she states, "but you are in no position to get up right now."

I clench my jaw as the two healthcare assistants take my trolley to an assessment room with sliding doors and close the blue curtains around it. While the HCAs are assisting me with taking off my clothes, my favourite tight jeans, and a warm sweater, I remember my grandma's advice on always wearing clean and hole-free undies. Luckily, I had clean G-strings on. Taking off my jeans, however, is a painful struggle.

As the HCAs gently help me undress, every move of my muscles causes renewed pain. I take deep breaths, trying to endure the discomfort because I don't want my favourite jeans to have to be cut off.

Once I am undressed, the HCAs put a blue hospital gown on me and have me lie on my left side. They place a cold metal bedpan beneath me, then roll me onto my back to use it. *How have I gone from having a normal Sunday morning to needing help to pee?*

"I can't do this," I tell one of the HCAs, feeling awkward.

"It's okay, just take a deep breath and try again," she says reassuringly.

I close my eyes and try to relax. I need to pee badly, but my brain won't let me. After a few moments, I open my eyes to find that I am alone in the room. A tap is running at a sink somewhere in the room, and the blue curtain is drawn around me. I pray silently, asking God for help. Finally, I feel the warmth of my urine trickling into the bedpan, and I sigh with relief.

When the HCAs come back into the room, they turn me onto my left side, remove the bedpan, and wipe me down. As they tend to me, I fight back tears. I feel utterly vulnerable. I go to church most Sundays and have always considered myself a strong believer. I've always felt great comfort in being able to ask God for help and feeling His presence through challenges I faced growing up, but this is something new.

Once they leave me alone, I start praying again, pleading with God to fix whatever is wrong with me so I can go home that night and maybe even get to work on Tuesday. I promise Him that I will take it easy if only He will make the pain go away.

As I am wheeled outside the private examination room and into the chaos of the crowded A&E department, I continue to implore God inwardly. The HCA asks the nurse where to park my trolley, and it ends up right next to the nursing station. It feels like a commando ops headquarters, with phones ringing incessantly and charts coming in and out.

I am keenly aware of all that is happening around me, and it is both distracting and overwhelming. While waiting for Anthony to arrive, I try to focus by jotting down notes in the notebook I carry in my purse. Writing has always been a way to centre my thoughts and feel in control.

My green whistle, a parting gift from the paramedic who brought me here, is a constant presence in my mouth. Its strong aftertaste and the fuzzy feeling it gives me are both comforting and disorienting. The pain is bearable when I lie flat, but any movement sends sharp waves of agony through my body.

A doctor checks on me briefly, and I force a smile, telling him I am okay. But the pain is getting worse, and I ask for another painkiller. The nurse has to consult with the doctor before giving me more. I have already taken a cocktail of drugs, but they are doing little to mask whatever my body is going through.

When Anthony finally arrives with our son Ryan, he is carrying a container of home-cooked food. The smell of roast chicken with gravy, broccoli, carrots, and potatoes makes my stomach growl. The nurse behind the desk looks our way and jokingly asks for some.

Anthony adjusts my trolley to be more upright, his movements careful and deliberate. Even this small motion sends a wave of pain through me, and I wince.

"Is that better, honey?" he asks, concern lacing his voice.

"A bit." I force a smile that I hope reassures him. "Thank you."

He brushes a strand of hair from my forehead. "I wish I could take this pain away."

Ryan sits at the end of the bed, swinging his legs nervously. His eyes are wide with a mixture of curiosity and fear.

"Mom, why did the game hurt you?" he asks, his voice small.

I take a deep breath, trying to manage the pain and my own emotions. "I'm not sure, sweetie. Sometimes things happen that we don't expect."

"The doctors are figuring it out, Ryan," Anthony tells him. "We'll know soon."

He turns back to me, concern evident in his eyes. "I'm sorry we took so long. I had to leave Collin at the boarding school first."

"How is he?"

My husband sighs, squeezing my hand. "He was worried about you. I talked with the boarding staff and asked them to keep an eye on him. They'll make sure he's not too stressed."

I nod. "Thank you for taking care of that. I know Collin can get anxious."

Ryan moves closer, his brow furrowed with concern. "Mom, you need to eat to get better."

I try to feed myself, but the pain is too much. A wave of nausea hits me. "I don't feel hungry anymore," I tell Anthony, feeling guilty that he brought such nice food all this way.

He takes the spoon from my hand. "That's okay. You don't have to eat right now."

Ryan reaches out and touches my arm lightly. "Mom, it's okay if you can't eat. We just want you to feel better."

I reach out and gently ruffle his hair. "I know, buddy. I will."

Anthony kisses my forehead softly. "Mommy is a fighter. She will get better soon."

The doctor strides down the hallway toward us. He stops in front of my trolley and announces, "I'm ready to examine you now." A nurse wheels me to a vacant room.

The doctor begins with a recap of my condition. "Do you experience incontinence?" he asks.

I'm not sure what that means, and he must see the confusion on my face. He elaborates, "Can you control your bowel movements?"

Embarrassed, I fumble for an answer, "I think so ... I mean, I don't need to use the bathroom right now." I must sound ridiculous to him, confused as to how my bowel movements might be related to my back injury. It must be important, since it's one of the first questions he asks.

The doctor signals for the nurse to come back into the room, and I struggle to keep up with their hurried conversation. Maybe it's the medication or the pain, but I find it hard to follow the exchange. They close the curtains around me, and the nurse helps me turn onto my side. I cry out. Just this small movement hurts so much.

"I'm sorry," the doctor murmurs, "I just need to check for rectal incontinence." Suddenly, I feel a finger probing my anus, and my muscles tense involuntarily. "Good news," he announces, removing his gloves, "you don't need emergency surgery."

My heart races at the mention of surgery. "Wait a minute," I stammer, "how can you tell I don't need surgery just by checking for incontinence? Don't you need to do an MRI or a scan?"

"If you had incontinence, it could indicate damage to your lumbar and sacral nerve roots," the doctor explains, "and that's a serious condition. Without surgery, you could become paralyzed."

The nurse rolls me back onto my back, and the pain comes roaring back. "I'm going to give you morphine intravenously," the doctor says, "to help relax your muscles and take away some of the pain." As the drug takes effect, my mind continues to race. How could a simple game of tug of war turn into something so serious?

But at least I don't need surgery. That news gives me a tad of relief.

Anthony is allowed into the examination room as the doctor writes on my chart and explains to the two of us that I have severely injured my back.

"It will take six weeks for your back to heal, your muscles to reknit, and those ligaments to strengthen," he announces.

I am stunned. "I can't stay away from work that long," I protest. "Maybe there's a shortcut, something else I could do?"

The doctor looks at me levelly. "Mrs. Roys, you need rest and physiotherapy to heal properly."

"Can't I just take a few days off?" I plead with him. "I promise I'll see my GP and get another certificate."

The doctor shakes his head. "I don't think you understand the severity of your injury." I try to argue again, but the doctor interrupts, asking, "After your fall last year, how long did it take for your toe to heal?"

I glance at my foot. "A few months." He gives a tight smile and explains that my toe could have healed faster if I had taken it easier. Tears well up in my eyes, and I wonder how I'm going to manage staying off work for so long.

The doctor continues, but my mind wanders, considering whether a quick fix is possible. Maybe he can give me stronger meds. Somehow, I'm not considering the fact that I'm lying flat on my back, unable to move without excruciating pain. I'm in no position to *not* listen to medical advice, but a small part of me (or perhaps a not-so-small part) wants to ignore him.

"I'm committed to my work," I tell him. "I don't like to leave things undone, but I'll see my GP, and he can give me another cert if I need it." The doctor agrees, though he seems reluctant, and gives me a five-day cert so I can see my GP.

He turns to my husband. "The nurses will call you when the intravenous meds take effect, so you can pick your wife up. It will likely be a few hours."

As the doctor leaves, the nurse wheels me outside to the nurses' station once more. The hospital is busy, and there's no space to move. But I'm determined that, by the time my husband returns, I will be able to stand on my feet and walk out of this place.

The morphine in my veins makes me feel light-headed. I try to pray, but it's impossible to focus on anything with the commotion all around me. Phones keep ringing. One nurse is scolding a doctor who just finished a 24-hour shift and discharged a patient with an IV still in his arm. A patient who reeks of alcohol keeps pestering the nurses at the station, asking to see a doctor. I'm just hoping no one will jostle my trolley and send another surge of pain through me.

I distract myself by trying to piece together the stories of the patients, focusing on faces I see in the corridor or spot in adjoining rooms. Many are elderly, sitting alone. I'm not the only one here, suffering. I watch the doctor interacting with an elderly man on a stretcher. His urine pouch is visible with a brown dark liquid in it. The doctor is explaining that he needs to be kept for further testing. He seems to not want to be in hospital. I don't blame him.

The hours pass with nurses checking on me from time to time, and they finally alert my husband that he can come collect me. The doctor discharges me with a referral for an MRI of my spine and a letter for my GP.

"Take care and do try to rest, Mrs. Roys," he says as he heads down the hallway, on to the next patient.

I am finally able to get up. I wobble out of the hospital *on my own two feet,* thanking God for this small miracle.

Chapter 4

Breakdown

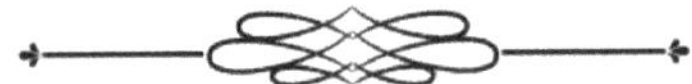

The stabbing pressure in my head is becoming unbearable. My thoughts are a chaotic mess, and I feel like I am drowning in a sea of emotions. Distractions are no longer working as the pain reaches around to my face, getting worse with each passing moment. A part of me wants to scream out in agony, but I try to keep a lid on it. I can't let anyone know how scared and vulnerable I feel.

It's a cold November night in the middle of a work week, and I am sitting on a very uncomfortable chair in the A&E waiting area of St. Vincent's Hospital, Dublin. The place is packed, and the noise level is high. The triage nurse gave me some painkillers earlier, when I first arrived, but they aren't doing much to ease the pain. I am on the urgent list, but due to a sudden influx of casualties from a nearby car accident, I have to wait. I try to remain calm, but the pain is starting to take over.

Aisling, a colleague and dear friend, keeps me company. She holds my black overcoat and MK purse while the triage nurse checks me and offers a gentle smile when I return. I sit down once more, feeling dizzy and disoriented. I am so grateful for Aisling's presence here. She had driven me to the care doctor earlier, and then to the hospital, even though I was dismissive of the need to go. Now, as I wait to see a doctor, she remains by my side, trying to help me find a comfortable position.

I close my eyes and try to rest my head on my overcoat, using Aisling's lap as a pillow. But the sharp pain in my face and head only intensifies. It feels like cold blood is flowing on the top of my head, and I can feel the pressure building up in my ear. Tears start streaming down my face, and I try to focus on breathing in and out just to keep in control.

The pain worsens. I look around at the other people in the waiting area, many of whom seem to be in worse condition than me. There's a young lad with a homemade bandage on his head, a lady who is high or drunk—possibly both—holding a throw-up bag, and a few elderly folks waiting in silence. I try to distract myself by guessing what their ailments might be, but the pain in my head is relentless.

"I can't focus on anything but the pain," I tell Aisling.

"Should we tell the nurse?" she asks. "They should know if it's getting worse."

I shake my head. I shouldn't be a priority when so many other people here need help. I consider going to the bathroom, which is only a few metres away, but the thought of the germs and smells is putting me off. *Never mind, I can hold it.*

I keep telling myself that I need to be strong, to keep it together. But the pain continues to increase and distractions are no longer working.

At last, a doctor calls my name. He leads the way to the examination room, his youthful face illuminated by the dim lights of the hospital room. His presence is a small comfort. As he begins to examine me, his fingers probing gently at my face, a shock of pain makes my whole body shudder.

"Can you follow my finger with one eye open, then the other?" he asks, his finger tracing a path from above my head to my chin and to the sides of my face. I follow his instructions, trying to ignore the constant burning in my face.

He remarks on how good my vision is, but as he touches my forehead, I flinch. My face is hypersensitive, and even the gentlest touch feels like an electric shock. I try to explain how I am feeling, but the words don't come out right.

"I'm probably just exhausted," I manage to say. "I've been working really hard, and I hurt my back not long ago, but I didn't slow down like my doctor suggested."

The doctor's brow furrows. "I think we need to do a CT scan to be sure. You'll need to stay overnight so we can monitor you and give you some stronger medication."

I have to spend the night in the hospital? I try to put on a brave face but am scared at what the CT scan might reveal.

As I walk back to Aisling, I glance around at patients in the cubicles nearby. They are all in the same boat, waiting anxiously for news from the doctors. I feel a pang of loneliness despite the presence of my friend.

"You can go home now," I tell her. "I have to stay overnight, but I'll be fine."

"I'm staying with you," she insists. "Until you're settled in your bed, at least." I'm secretly grateful for her company. My family is too far away to offer comfort right now.

As I wait for a bed to become available, I recall the panic I felt as I texted my husband a few hours ago. "On the way to hospital with a suspected minor stroke. Aisling is taking me, and phone battery low, but I will be fine."

My husband called immediately after receiving my text, and Aisling was keeping him abreast of my situation. Now, in a cold hospital waiting room, more than two hours away from home, all I want is the comfort of my husband's arms around me. I know it's impractical. He's home with the boys where he needs to be, but part of me wishes he would find a way to drive through this cold November night, push open the hospital doors, and just be with me.

I can't shake the thought that I am a burden to everyone around me. Aisling had to pay exorbitant fees for parking. I know she has a ton of stuff to do at work, yet she insisted on staying with me into the wee hours of the night. I feel the weight of my disruption on her and on my family as well.

I try to hold back my tears, but the pain is relentless. I'd gone through and sacrificed so much to make it to this point, it feels unfair to be faced with this now.

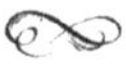

My stress levels were through the roof during the last two years of my university studies. Something had to give, though it took me a while to realize it. It wasn't until a deep conversation with Anthony that it hit me. He pointed out that I was barely home, sometimes arriving as late as 11 p.m.

He was right. I had been trying to fit everything in, but things were slipping through the cracks—the things I loved and cared about the most—my family. The university library had become my home away from home. I would leave the house at 6:45 a.m. to hit the gym by 7:00 and swim or exercise before starting work at 8:00 a.m.

Somehow, I had been keeping all the balls in the air. I'd remained at the top of my class, maintained my marriage, and navigated my kids' struggles through school.

When my son wasn't allowed to speak in class due to answering all the questions, because he was apparently "too smart," I was livid. Yes, he learned to read by age three. Yes, he had a mother who had studied early education and pedagogy. I had given him flashcards, math dot programs, and countless opportunities for performing and communicating from a very early age. I moved him from the local school to an all-Irish school to keep him challenged and engaged.

It wasn't easy to come home to an eight-year-old crying about his day, feeling misunderstood and silenced in class. He was a communicator who loved to talk and couldn't keep quiet. As a mother, it felt like my heart was being crushed. Was I abandoning my duties as a mother in pursuit of a piece of paper?

I cried many nights when I lay in bed wondering, *what is this all for?* I had to remind myself I was doing all of this to give my boys a better future, to show them that they could achieve whatever goals they set for themselves. But I felt completely drained.

After that talk with my husband, I started dropping my boys off at school on my way to the university so I could spend some time with them, which meant I had to cut back on exercise. I made it a point to be home for dinner at 6 p.m. After dinner and a little time with the kids, I would put them to bed by 7:30 or 8:00 and then be back at it. Studying my books, answering emails, coordinating nursing home visits, or sorting through volunteer applications—interviewing and vetting people before they could visit the nursing homes.

Things grew more stressful when my husband started a master's program during my final year. Why not? I was already studying; he could study too, and we continued our juggling act.

A relentless drive had helped me push open doors that might have held me back. But now I was here, my back against a wall and no exit door in sight.

At 4 a.m., a bed is finally available, and I'm taken through darker corridors of the A&E department. The place is packed, with trolleys and people lining the hallway. I spot some familiar faces—people I had seen earlier in the waiting area, including the lady who looked high and an elderly gentleman who was holding his nose with a handkerchief. He's sleeping in a chair while I get a bed, and I feel guilty for taking it.

Aisling finally agrees to leave, but not until she's sure I've been given medication. I'm given one for my stomach and another one intravenously, along with a drip. It will take a while for the meds to take effect, but I'm grateful for the small relief they bring.

The nurse who helps me get settled in is from the Philippines, and his bubbly personality is a nice distraction from the chaos around me. I listen to the machines and monitors beeping around me. There are at least five hospital beds in this small room, each of us separated by blue curtains, with a nurse station at the entrance. People are moaning and groaning in pain, and the green light above my head is the only source of light in the room.

I try to hold back my tears, but they come streaming anyway. I cry as quietly as I can, feeling lonely and scared. So many questions run through my mind. *Why does it feel like my face is being cut with fiery jolts? What's with the burning on the right side of my face, near my cheek and jaw?* The pressure in my head feels like a balloon slowly filling up with air, getting ready to burst. I try to keep my breathing steady and not let panic take over.

The medication finally kicks in, and my back feels normal for the first time in a very long time. I've been going about with this back injury for so long, I couldn't remember what it felt like to have absolutely no back pain!

Yet the pain in my head and the jolts of pain across my face have not faded. It is weird that the medication doesn't make a difference to this. *What is going on with my body?*

Chapter 5

This Can't Be Happening

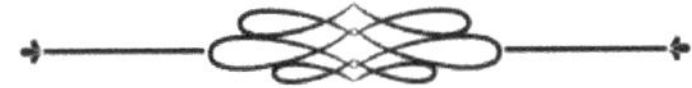

A hospital is not the most comfortable place to sleep. Understatement of the year. Despite being exhausted and finally crying myself to sleep, I keep waking due to the constant noise from the nurses and HCAs. As day breaks, the noise in the corridor increases with the changing of shifts and the start of patient rounds.

I feel groggy and heavy, with dizzy spells. The jolts of pain on my face continue intermittently, while numbness and burning sensations on the bottom half of my face are a constant. I pray for strength and grace because I need to leave the hospital soon; I have plans, my younger sister is arriving tonight from Brazil, and I have a whole itinerary for her brief visit. Activities that don't involve being in hospital!

As I wait in line to use the bathroom, the lady in front of me, who I'd spoken to the night before, starts telling me about her husband's heart surgery. We chat for a while, and I feel comforted by her company. It reminds me once more that I am not the only one facing uncertainty.

After my turn in the bathroom, I quickly wash my hands and face and return to my bed. A porter waits for me with a wheelchair.

"I can walk," I insist, but he tells me to get in the chair, something about it being regulation. As he wheels me down the corridor, I feel terribly self-conscious. But I am more concerned about the pain on the side of my head, which is increasing with each moment.

My phone rings, and as soon as I see my boss' name on caller ID, I answer. "Good morning, Michele, how are you feeling today?" he asks in his usually upbeat tone of voice.

"I'm okay. Waiting on a scan in the hospital, but I think I'm just tired." I try to hold back my worries and concerns and keep a businesslike tone of voice. "Were you able to look over the latest candidate interview I left on your desk?"

He lets out an incredulous laugh. "Michele, you're in the hospital. Forget about work and focus on *you* for once." He is right. While here, I told myself I would not worry about work, but it's almost impossible given my packed work schedule.

"Okay, I'll try."

"Great, keep me updated and please forget about this place. Just focus on getting better." He ends the call.

In the CT scan room, a nurse helps me onto the stretcher-like bed. It's my first time having a CT scan. I don't want it to reveal anything too serious, but I hope it will reveal *something*. I want answers to this constant pain.

The machine is round like a donut, and as it begins to take pictures of my head, a cold breeze sweeps across the room, causing more pain on my right side. I am relieved when the nurse returns less than five minutes later to say it's over.

As the porter takes me back down the hallways, I wonder what the results will reveal. "I hope it's nothing serious," I mutter as I am wheeled back to the safety of the little bed.

The pain and shocks still linger. It's like a never-ending nightmare I'm stuck in. I can't shake it off, and I don't know what *it* is—besides unsettling, unnerving ... and driving me insane.

As I wait for the consultant to return, I strike up a conversation with a fellow patient. His parents were with him last night, and they looked worried sick. He tells me that he fell and hit his head while on his college campus, and he doesn't remember much about it. He initially refused to go with the ambulance. I can understand why. A college student, he probably had a bit too much to drink. We chat for a while, and again I feel the relief of getting my mind off my own pain and uncertainty, at least for a few moments.

While getting the scan done, I missed breakfast, but the kind HCA offers me tea and toast. I'm grateful for this small comfort. The warm cup in my hands and the aroma of fresh tea with a dash of milk help ease my mind during the long wait.

My dizzy spells have lessened, but the right side of my face still feels heavy, and I have itching, crawling sensations like ants on my skin. It's not as severe as before. Maybe it's getting better. Maybe thinking positively will reverse anything bad that could happen to me.

My phone's battery is low, so I head down the corridor to find the charging station. The porter tells me the way out and advises me to show my wristband to the security guard. As I walk down the corridor, I see the lady whose husband had a heart attack the previous night. She tells me he had surgery and is now waiting for a bed. She hugs me, and I feel the relief in her embrace. We're complete strangers, but there's a deeper connection between us, a sense of camaraderie and vulnerability that only a hospital can bring out.

As I step outside into the A&E waiting area, I see a pregnant woman in a lot of pain. She was here last night and was discharged but came back this morning. I send up a prayer for her, put my phone in the charger, and head back to my cubicle.

I can't rest. The sterile smell of the hospital, the machines beeping, the rush all around me—all these increase my feeling of trepidation as I lie on the hospital bed.

The consultant walks towards me, charts in hand, looks at me over his glasses, and asks me to describe my symptoms again. He conducts his own examination, carefully avoiding the right side of my face which is hyper-sensitive. It still feels sensitive and numb at the same time, with the razor-like pain across my face that brought me here with the concern that I might be having a stroke.

After about 15 minutes, he is ready to give his verdict. I hold my breath.

"The good news is that it doesn't seem to be a stroke or a tumour causing the pain." He pauses and places the chart beside him. "This episode seems more related to trigeminal neuralgia. I will be referring you to a neurologist to help you going forward."

"What is trigeminal neuralgia?" Even forming those words is a tongue twist for me.

"It is a pain disorder connected with the three branches of your facial nerve coming from the V cranial nerve on the brain stem," he explains.

"How did I get it?" I ask. "Can you be certain of this diagnosis?"

"It's not well understood, but it can be caused by a blood vessel pressing on the nerve or other underlying conditions, which can cause intense facial pain. From the scan, we have ruled out the first two possibilities: aneurysm or tumour. It's unlikely to be MS which can also cause this type of pain, so it could likely be a virus." He looks down once again at his chart. "I'm going to write you a prescription for pain medication."

I can't help but feel a sense of disappointment, "So you don't know for sure what's causing this pain, and you don't know how to cure it?"

"Unfortunately, that's the nature of this condition," he replies. "But the neurologist will be able to help manage your pain and work with you to find the best course of treatment."

"But what about my face? Why is it still feeling heavy and numb, yet everything is very heightened? Is this part of trigeminal neuralgia?" I am not at all happy with this news.

"Mrs. Roys," the consultant says in a gentle tone, "each person has a different reaction and what might suit one person might not suit another. Not everyone with trigeminal neuralgia feels numbness, but the pain and shocks you've described are very much in line with this condition."

"When will I get better?" I have to know.

He hesitates. "I can't say how long it will take for your face to return to normal. It can be weeks, months, or in some cases years."

Years? But it's his next words that hit me sideways.

"In any case, you need to listen to your body."

Listen to my body? How do I even do that? I've lived with the "mind over matter" motto for years now. I have no idea how to change that part of me.

The consultant hands me a few papers. "Here is your prescription for pain medication, a certificate for you to give to your workplace and also to your GP. Please see the neurologist as soon as you can."

I read through his cert for work. "I can't afford to take more time off. I've already scheduled four days off work this week. That should be enough. This certificate states I need four *weeks* with a review!" I'm sure the frustration is evident in my tone of voice.

"I am sorry, Mrs. Roys, but you need to rest and allow your body to settle. I am suggesting four weeks, but to be honest I think you will need a lot more time off work. This is a painful and potentially chronic condition, and you still need to find the right medication to help you."

Is he for real? "Can you please give me a cert for a few days instead? I can go to my GP if I need it to be extended." He reluctantly agrees to my pleading.

"I have another appointment, but please mind yourself Mrs. Roys." I note the sympathy in his voice. His eyes, though tired, show concern and care, which I am grateful for.

"Thank you," I manage to say, clutching the papers.

I try to recall everything he told me. Weeks? Years? I have a full schedule at work—issues to resolve for the employees, labour court cases to prepare, recruitment drives to fill, and a new human resources management system to launch for the whole company.

There's no way I need that much time off work just for my face to go back to normal. Maybe after my four-day holiday, everything will be sorted out. I'll prove to the doctor that I can heal from trigeminal neuralgia in no time. This illness is not part of my plan.

I call Aisling. My friend already stayed with me most of the night and now she has to pick me up. On the drive from the hospital, she suggests that I stay at her house instead of returning to my rented room.

"It would make me sleep better knowing you're not on your own," she says. I feel like an inconvenience to her. To everyone.

The worst part isn't the pain, the burning sensation, or the crawling-ants-inside-my-head feeling. It is the loss of control, not being able to tell my body to obey, to just stop hurting already and heal itself. I can't go to work. I can't drive myself home. My husband will need to come to Dublin by bus to pick up my car, which I left at work, and then drive me home.

I leave the hospital with a diagnosis but no answers. Only more questions.

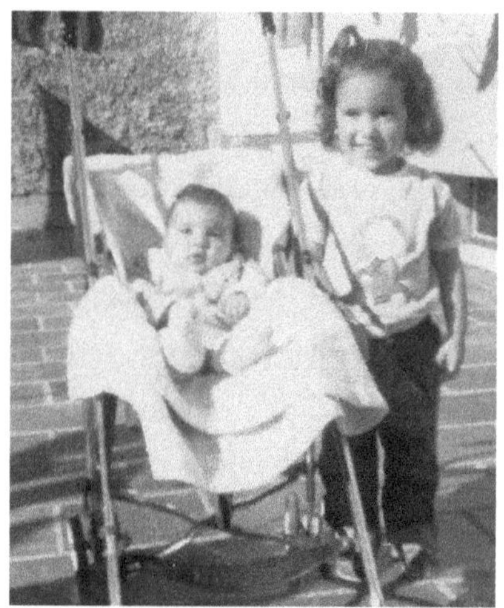

Caxias do Sul - RS- Brazil

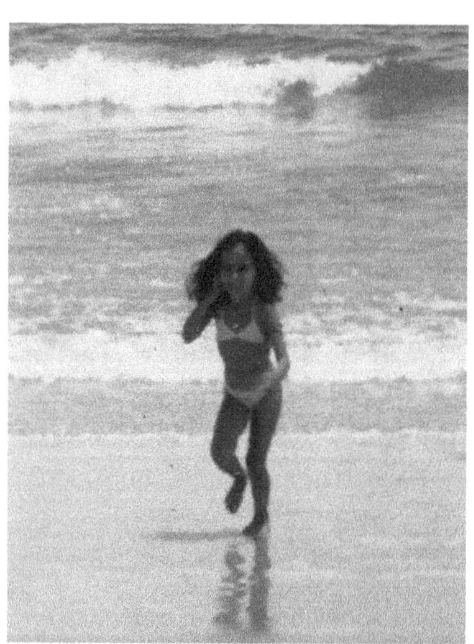

Florianopolis -SC- Brazil

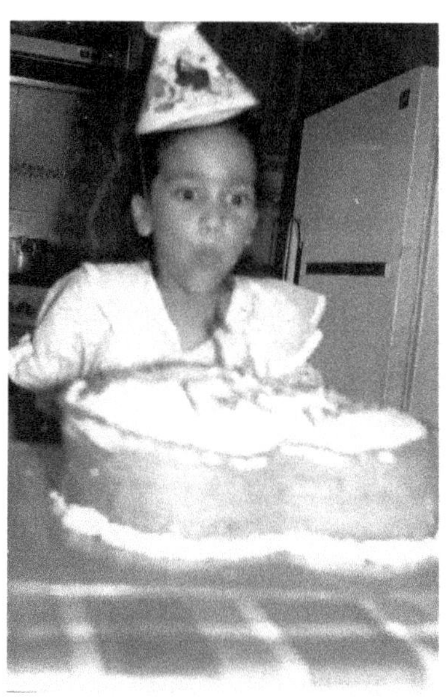

Campo Grande - MG - Brazil

Part 2: Denial

"The attempt to escape from pain, is what creates more pain."
– **Gabor Maté**

Chapter 6

Diagnosis

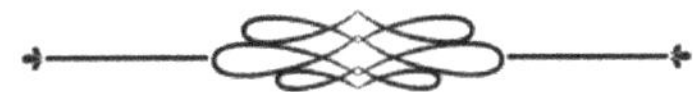

I'm sitting in my living room, wrapped in a blue blanket. A fire crackles in the fireplace, casting a warm, flickering glow on the room. The warmth does nothing to ease the pain that grips my face, alternating between a strange numbness and zaps of lightning pain. I shift in my chair, trying to find a comfortable position, but it's no use. The pressure in my head, as if it's about to explode, doesn't wane.

My pen moves across the pages of my well-worn journal, documenting the turmoil I feel inside. One question keeps arising in my mind. *Why?* Followed by another question. *When will it stop?* It's been a month already!

I'm a Type-A personality, always on the go, always productive, always in control. But now, I'm forced to stop working and my whole world feels upside down. It's frightening being pushed into this situation after I'd been spending so much time away from home, focused on my work commitments.

When I was well, I didn't spend as much time with my family as I should have. I wasn't there for my eldest son, Collin, navigating secondary school and its challenges. I wasn't available to help my youngest son, Ryan, with his homework or to read with him before bed. I've spent so little time with Anthony face to face lately and hardly know how he's coping with his work or what his struggles have been. Now, they are the only ones showing up for me. Guilty isn't a strong enough word for how I feel.

The first two weeks after my release from the hospital with the tentative diagnosis of trigeminal neuralgia were the hardest. Learning how to deal with a constant, invisible pain feels like I've been given the task of taming a wild beast.

But my greatest struggle is settling that part of me that wants control and answers, and is angry for not getting either. I thought I was invincible, but now I'm reminded that my body can stop, and it has.

Now that my life has screeched to a sudden halt, I feel the storm brewing inside. The invincible persona who held it all together on the outside is gone. Will the storm reveal that all I've built is a house of cards? In my journal, I make a list of words to describe how I feel: *helpless, incapable, vulnerable, unworthy, a burden, a weight, a fraud.*

I look fine, and that makes it even worse. I see myself in the mirror and my mind can't seem to grasp the fact that I am in pain with some kind of invisible illness, and nothing can be done about it.

I don't know what to do with myself, and I don't know how to deal with my condition. Although my husband and sons have rallied around me, I feel alone. No one understands what I am going through.

This sudden switch in my day-to-day life has been torturous. I'm used to being on the go. Now, I have no energy. Constant pain drains me. I journal question after question. *Will I ever be able to go back to work? Will I have to find a new career? What kind of work can a woman with an invisible illness even do?*

I try to keep busy listening to audiobooks, podcasts, guided meditations, but the pain and fatigue make it hard for me to focus on anything. I am stuck in a loop of pain and rest, pain and rest, with energy for little else.

But as I sit here, wrapped in my blue blanket, with the fire crackling in the background, I scribble in my journal a few things that bring me hope. *I am not alone. I have my family. The neurologist might help me find a way to manage the pain. There is hope I will be able to live my life to the fullest—somehow.*

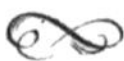

The December air is crisp and biting as I step out of my husband's car, my face pulled tight with pain.

"I'll pick you up in an hour," he says.

"Okay, thanks." I close the passenger door, but frustration edges my thoughts as I make my way up the long, narrow pathway of an Edwardian home.

Tall, thin houses on either side loom over me, their metal gates glinting in the dreary winter light, as I approach a dark green door.

I take a deep breath to steady my nerves. I'm here to seek help, but the thought of talking to a stranger about my pain and uncertainty fills me with dread, even if she is a therapist. I knock three times as a cold breeze sweeps through my hair.

The door opens and I am greeted by a slight woman with dark hair and a warm smile. "Welcome, Michele." The therapist introduces herself as Rose as she shows me in.

Warmth from the fireplace envelops me, and I detect the fragrant aroma of cinnamon and orange. Angel decorations adorn the living room and large, delicate statues surround a beautifully decorated Christmas tree. The fireplace is the centrepiece of the room, its cosy blaze casting a warm glow over the space. Tall drapes on the windows are from a different era, adding a sense of nostalgia to the charming ambiance of the home.

Rose gestures for me to take a seat on the brown leather couch opposite her. I shrug off my jacket and remove my hat, scarf, and gloves, trying to make myself comfortable. As I look around the living room, I notice family photos on the mantelpiece, giving the home a personal touch.

I take a deep breath, and the scent of cinnamon and orange offer a sense of calm and tranquillity. Yet as Rose invites me to tell her more about myself, I can't shake the feeling of hopelessness at my situation.

"To say I feel apprehensive is an understatement," I begin, feeling a tremor in my voice as I try to get my emotions in check. "I've already been to four doctors, and the pain is only getting worse. I don't know when, or if, I'll ever get better."

"What is the hardest thing for you right now?" she asks.

"I just want a quick fix," I say. "I don't want to spend months or even years in therapy."

"I understand." Rose nods in empathy. "But healing and finding solutions isn't always a quick process."

I sigh. I know she is right, but I'd much prefer immediate answers and solutions.

As we go through paperwork and discuss the reasons for my seeking help, she tells me this is a confidential session. She explains that she will need to evaluate my mood. "If you are at risk or suicidal, I will have to break the confidentiality agreement and get a third party to intervene."

"I reject the idea of suicide," I tell her, hoping my certainty is clear in my voice. "Yes, I'm confused and yes, I'm in a lot of pain, but I know how precious life is and the repercussions of ending my life, the toll it would have on my family and children. You don't need to worry about that."

I just want to be back to my former, busy, accomplished and sure self, but it feels like that woman is slipping further and further away. Rose listens, but her words of sympathy and encouragement only frustrate me. I don't want her understanding; I want a cure.

As Rose starts to speak again, I try to focus, but my mind races with thoughts of my diagnosis: trigeminal neuralgia, a rare and painful disease that affects the trigeminal nerve, the nerve responsible for sensation in the face. I force the thoughts aside.

"Michele, I understand that you are feeling a lot of frustration and anger right now. It's understandable that you want a quick fix and to be healed as soon as possible. But healing and recovery are not linear. It's important for us to work through your feelings to help you understand the root of your pain."

I nod, but inside I am seething. I don't want to talk about my feelings.

"I know it's difficult." Rose seems to sense my reluctance. "But discussing your emotions will help you better cope with your condition. It's also important for us to talk about the impact this has on your relationships, namely with your husband and children."

I sigh again. She is right. I have seen the way my husband and children are struggling to adjust to seeing me in pain and not being able to help. In the month since my diagnosis, the strain on our family has grown apparent.

"It's vital for us to work through this together," Rose continues. "We will also consider ways for you to manage your pain and cope with the uncertainty and changes in your life."

I nod, letting resignation wash over me. It joins the frustration that has already made itself at home in my mind.

We schedule the next appointment, and I step out into the cold December afternoon. A small sense of hope appears, pushing its way between the looming emotions of frustration and resignation. This won't be easy, but I am willing to do whatever it takes to get my life back and be there for my family.

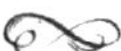

As I sit in Rose's living room for the third time this month, I note the holiday decor but feel distant from the festive season. The pain is overwhelming, and it seems like no one understands. I try to express my fears to Rose.

"Can this be psychosomatic?" The words get caught in my throat as I struggle to hold back tears.

"Take your time," she assures me.

I take a deep breath to compose myself. "I have doctors validating my illness, but what if they are wrong? Maybe there is something internal that I can find and deal with that will make the pain disappear. Is that possible?" I want her to help me find the root problem in the next four sessions we have scheduled, so I can deal with it and everything can go back to normal.

Rose looks at me with a gentle smile. I wonder if she took a class on this: Compassionate Expressions 101. Her words do little to ease my turmoil. "I'm sorry you are feeling this way. It must be very hard for you. You might feel like no one understands, even your family."

It's nothing I haven't already heard. Her words fade into the background as I gaze out the tall windows. No one has an answer for me. This is the harsh reality; I must figure it out on my own.

"Maybe you have not accepted that your health has made you stop." A change in Rose's tone brings me back into the conversation. "The more you try to struggle to get back to normal, the more your body will fight with you because you haven't actually learned to listen to it."

This statement resonates. I tend to ignore my body signals, even the different accidents I had leading up to this point. In each instance, I bulldozed through the pain and injuries. But this time, regardless of how much I try, my body is not cooperating.

I feel defeated. I am exhausted, in constant pain, and the new medication I was prescribed has only made things worse. I can't do even the smallest things. Even making my bed exhausts me. I get my side of the sheets straightened and then have to rest so I can get the other half done!

Is it so wrong to want a quick fix? Is there something my body is trying to tell me? If so, can't it use a language other than pain? I should be fluent by now but still can't understand a word.

Chapter 7

Emotional Resistance

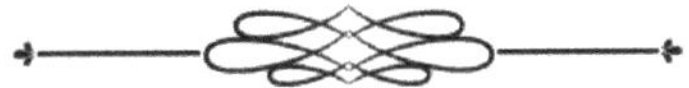

The cosy fire in my living room provides a stark contrast to the bitter weather outside. It is the outdoors that mirror the turmoil in my mind. "Mom, why can't you get a glass of water yourself?" My son's offhand comment echoes in my mind.

I can't shake off the expression of disappointment that washed over my husband's face when he arrived home to find me still in my pyjamas, lost in my thoughts and trying to hold back tears. I turn to my journal, the one companion that seems to truly understand me.

Today marks three months since my diagnosis of trigeminal neuralgia, a journey as rough as this persistent physical pain. Numbness on the right side of my face, heaviness, pins and needles on the extremities of my face, pain in my jaw, temple, and forehead, stiffness in my neck, and increasing pain in my lower back and legs are all constant companions.

"It's an invisible illness," I explain to my friends and family, trying to make them understand why I look the same as ever but am struggling inside.

Somehow, the emotional pain is even worse than the physical pain, especially when well-meaning friends and acquaintances ask, "How come you're still ill? You look just fine." It is a comment I've heard too many times, and my sense of self-worth dwindles every time I try to come up with an answer.

As a mother, I feel like a failure, unable to go hiking and have adventures with my boys like I used to. Instead of playing catch with them in the yard, I watch them from the window, feeling disconnected from their joy. As a wife, I can barely manage intimacy with my husband, who remains my pillar. The basic chores of cleaning and cooking take all my energy, leaving me feeling inadequate and guilty as he picks up the slack without complaint.

I've become reclusive, avoiding meetups with my friends because I never know how I'll feel from one day to the next. I miss the laughter and camaraderie but hate having to cancel plans due to pain. Invitations to gatherings and parties have dwindled, and I feel a growing sense of isolation.

As a daughter, I should be the one caring for my aging mother, yet she's the one visiting and taking care of me. The roles have reversed, and I hate having her worry about me when she should be enjoying her golden years.

I've always been the strong, reliable one who listens and helps my siblings, but right now I don't have the bandwidth or brainpower to navigate family dynamics. I used to be the mediator and the shoulder to cry on, but now I can't even handle a phone call without feeling overwhelmed.

Small tasks around the house that I used to take for granted now seem impossible. *I need to do something productive.* I head to the messy bathroom and stand in the doorway, feeling overwhelmed at the thought of cleaning, an activity that used to be a breeze. I enjoyed putting things in order. *Mind over matter,* I tell myself.

I grab a sponge and start on the sink. Every swipe feels like I'm lifting weights. I manage to clean the mirror, but the pain hits hard when I move to the shower. I lean against the cool tiles, trying to breathe. I just can't do it. I make my way to the couch and collapse, my husband's worried eyes on me. As I sink into the cushions, I feel the weight of exhaustion pulling me down.

The front door swings open and my boys burst in, full of energy and stories from their day. My youngest hands me his homework, his eyes bright with expectation. I want to help him, to dive into his world of math problems and spelling tests, but the pain fogs my mind, making it hard to focus.

My eldest starts to talk about an argument with his friends, his tone edged with frustration. I try to listen, to be there for him, but each word feels like a sharp jab, making it hard to concentrate.

"I'm sorry, sweetie. I just need a moment," I say, forcing a smile that doesn't reach my eyes. Their disappointment is clear, and it adds to the heavy guilt I carry.

"I'm sorry, I can't make it." I text a response to my sister, cancelling yet another social event. I feel like I am failing everyone, and it only adds to my stress.

I want to find the root of my pain and make it go away. Rose tells me it doesn't work like that. "Acceptance is key," she has said several times. Each time, I wanted to scream. She tells me I haven't fully accepted my illness and that struggling to get back to normal is only making things worse.

How does one simply "accept" an illness of any kind, even more so an invisible one?

I try to take her advice and listen to my body—to accept my limitations, my fatigue, my weakness. But what I really want is to be the strong, capable woman I used to be. It was how I defined myself for so long, and I no longer know who I am.

The setting sun shines through the living room windows, but I barely notice it. I sit on the edge of the couch, my hands twisting nervously in my lap, as the familiar ache in my face and body intensifies. The soft cracking of the fireplace is a small comfort in an otherwise overwhelming day.

"I don't know what to do," I confess to my husband, my voice trembling as tears trickle down my face, blurring my vision. My chest feels tight.

His arms wrap around me, steady and warm. I bury my face in his shoulder, feeling his shirt dampening with my tears.

"I feel so lost, so helpless," I sob, my voice muffled against his chest. The familiar scent of his cologne is both comforting and heartbreaking, a reminder of the normalcy that feels so far away.

"We'll get through this," he whispers, his voice steady and soothing. He gently strokes my hair. "You're not alone, and we will find a way."

I nod, though I don't believe it. The pain is all-consuming, and it feels like there's no end in sight.

"I wish I could do more," I whisper, my voice barely audible. "I wish I could be the wife and mother you all deserve."

He pulls back slightly, just enough to look into my eyes. "You are a fighter, Michele. We will get through this."

I have to find a way to cope with the pain, both physically and emotionally, for my family if nothing else. But how do I find acceptance, much less learn to cope, when I am in a battle with my own mind and body? How do I reconcile the person I once was with the person I am now?

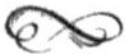

At 17, I was a small yet fierce brunette filled with inner strength and unshakeable belief. Barely over 1.5 meters tall, but with a desire to change the world.

A unique journey had begun two years earlier, on a serene Sunday morning. I was lounging by the poolside of my home in Brazil, flipping through a magazine as the sun warmed my skin.

Suddenly, a headline leapt off the page: "Come to India. We Need Help." The words resonated deeply. Goosebumps prickled my arms, and I felt an undeniable pull, as if God was speaking to me.

Right there, under the blue sky, I prayed fervently. "God, if this is Your will, make a way. I don't know how to do this, but I'm committed." That moment of clarity set my heart ablaze with purpose. I knew I had to go to India to help the children in need.

Two years of relentless determination followed. I navigated a labyrinth of bureaucratic hurdles, yet my resolve remained. My parents were divorced, with my legal father in Japan and my mother in southern Brazil. I lived with friends in São Paulo, where I tirelessly fundraised for my mission. Scepticism and doubt from friends and family only fuelled my resolve. I clung to my calling, refusing to be swayed.

The paperwork process was gruelling. My father had to travel six hours by train to the Brazilian Embassy in Tokyo multiple times, each trip met with new bureaucratic demands, to help me get the necessary paperwork together. My mother, too, made several trips to government offices, but obtaining the necessary documents seemed like a never-ending saga.

One sweltering afternoon, my mother and I made our way to a bustling shopping centre in Sao Paulo, clutching a stack of documents. The air was thick with humidity, and sweat trickled down my back as we navigated the crowded streets. We had an appointment to get my passport and request special permission from the Court of Minors for me to travel alone as a minor.

My father had already signed the necessary forms, emphatically stating he wouldn't make another trip to Tokyo. The weight of the documents in my hands felt like gold—invaluable and irreplaceable. However, we were only able to get my passport done that day. My mother returned home to be with my younger siblings, leaving me to tackle the final hurdle on my own.

A few days before my planned departure date, I made my way downtown. Desperation and determination intertwined as I navigated São Paulo's sprawling cityscape, taking three buses and walking through unfamiliar neighbourhoods, asking directions each step of the way for my journey of over two and half hours.

Finally, I arrived at the imposing building of the Court of Minors (Juizado de Menores). My heart pounded as I approached the reception desk, dwarfed by the towering architecture. I explained my situation to the receptionist, and she called for a legal assistant. Moments later, I found myself recounting my story once again.

"I need the judge's signature to travel to India in three days," I pleaded.

The assistant's eyes narrowed. "These things take months. There's a procedure," he explained, shaking his head.

"But I've been trying for years," I insisted. "I've faced countless delays, and I'm so close. Can you plead my case?"

He finally agreed to try. I waited, praying silently. *God, if you want me in India, you have to do this.*

Eventually, he returned and led me through a maze of corridors and up a flight of stairs. He opened a door, revealing the judge's office. "You have five minutes," he said, closing the door behind me.

The judge looked up as I entered, his gaze stern. "Thank you for seeing me," I began, trying to find my voice. "I'm going to India as a missionary, and all I need now is your signature to travel."

The judge leaned back in his chair, scrutinizing me. "Do you understand the gravity of your request? Human trafficking is a serious concern. You're only 17, traveling to another continent alone. Your father is in Japan, your mother is in southern Brazil, and you're here alone. Even to come to this office, at least one parent is usually present with the child. You're the first one seeking permission on your own!"

"I understand," I replied. "But how many people do you meet who have a calling from God to go to another country to help others? Would you want to stand in the way of what God is doing, or would you want to be part of it?"

He studied me for a moment, then sighed. "This is highly irregular. Do you realize the responsibility you're asking me to take on? You're a minor, and this is not a decision I can make lightly."

"I know it's a lot to ask," I said, feeling more certain than ever that this is what I was meant to do. "But I've faced so many obstacles and overcome each one. This is my calling, and I need your help to fulfil it."

The judge's expression softened slightly. "You've shown remarkable determination," he admitted, "but this decision could have serious implications."

I took a deep breath. "I understand the risks, but I also understand my purpose. God has no hands or feet, but ours, and I am willing to use mine to help those poor people like Mother Teresa. Please, help me make this journey possible."

After a long pause, he reached for his pen, signed the document, and handed it to me. "Take this downstairs and get it processed before I change my mind."

I thanked him profusely and practically flew out of the office, my heart soaring. The assistant helped me complete the process, and I left with the precious piece of paper in hand, another milestone reached in my journey to India.

At that moment, I knew that nothing could stop me if God was on my side.

Chapter 8

Introspection

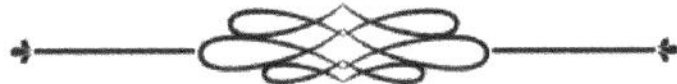

I sit on the circular brown couch in my room, wrapped in a white and pink bathrobe. Four months have passed, and I thought this nightmare would be over by now. Small things bother me. The smell of medicinal cream. The loud ticking of the wall clock. They all add to the hopelessness I feel at time passing by and leaving me stuck here in this place.

What have I done wrong? Why can't my body just work with me instead of against me? I pick up my journal and begin to vent my frustrations.

"Why can't you just fix yourself?" I scribble onto the pages. Today's pain is unbearable, but I have no choice except to bear it. Anger and frustration have become my constant, unwanted companions. I am angry at my body and frustrated at this trigeminal neuralgia.

"I can't do this anymore," I write, blinking back tears so they don't stain the pages of my journal. They stream down my face anyway. Something else that refuses to listen to me. I decide to write a letter to my invisible illness.

"You are annoying," I begin. "I would have never thought you would still be around after 4 MONTHS, reminding me of your ability to cause me to come to a complete stop! If I don't listen, your persuasive power brings me to my knees. But worse than the physical pain is how people can't see the torment you cause me. You are invisible to them, yet your venom controls me.

"I'm constantly struggling to put you out of my mind, suppressing you through deep breathing, meditation, and every tactic possible. But it's like trying to hold back a raging river. You have stripped me of my energy, my control, my ability to think and make things happen. I am not a fraction of the person I used to be. It feels like my body is a prison."

As I place my pen down, I feel somewhat better for having vented my feelings. I'm also exhausted. All I want is to sleep. I'm still mad, but in the space created by journaling, I find a thread of possibility.

Maybe I will regain my strength, even if it comes very slowly.

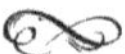

I sit in yet another waiting room. After ten minutes of waiting at the occupational health practice, a tall doctor walks in with a blue chart in hand. "Mrs. Michele Roys?" I gather my purse, scarf, and gloves, following him out of the waiting room into the second door on the left.

The doctor sits on a black office chair, his back to the window, and motions me to take a seat opposite him. As he pulls a pen from his shirt pocket, he asks, "Can you describe to me what has happened to you in as much detail as you can?"

I describe the last four months, the incident that led me to St. Vincent's Hospital that cold night, and what it's been like since.

"I feel terrible for still being sick," I finish.

"Have you been keeping a pain log?" the doctor asks.

"I've tried, but I don't want to think about my pain, where it is, the frequency, and the intensity. I feel that by recording it, I'm giving it more power to carve a pathway in my brain." I wipe away the tears stealing down my face.

The doctor listens intently. However, my level of pain today is high, and I can't do as much talking as I want to. He asks me about my c-sections, any other illnesses I've had, and my background. I explain about my type A personality, which I think is a huge factor, as slowing down and trying to take it easy is not happening for me.

Finally, I can sense that he's ready to give me his opinion. "Mrs. Roys, I am sorry you are in so much pain. The good news is that this is benign, but the bad news is that we don't know when you will get better. Everyone is different and reacts differently. I think your upcoming consultation with the neurologist will shed more light on the situation."

He pauses, perhaps looking for the right words. "Maybe you need to learn to slow down, take it easy, and allow your body to get better in its time."

I clench my jaw, angry at his suggestion. Did he not hear all I've just said?

My inner perfectionism screams, *More of this? What kind of answer is that anyway?* I try to silence the inner debate by asking the doctor more questions, but I am crushed by his suggestion to go slow. What does he think I've been doing for the last four months?

"When do you think I will be well enough to return to work?"

After a long silence, he answers, "I am sorry, but in my opinion, you are unfit for work for the foreseeable future." The doctor lowers his gaze.

Unfit. Foreseeable future. Each word is a straight punch to my face! The blows reverberate throughout my whole body as if I'm in a boxing ring. *Unfit. Slow down. Relax. Foreseeable future.* The hits just keep on coming.

I burst into tears. I am embarrassed to be crying in his office, but I can't help it. A snail can move faster than me. It's not like I don't already know I am unfit for work. Hell, I've been living with pain 24/7. Trigeminal neuralgia doesn't even rest for the Sabbath. Medications are useless and I am getting fed up with the side effects of drowsiness, mood swings, constipation, brain fog, weight gain, and dizzy spells!

I've been following every suggestion and doing everything I can to get better—in turns attempting to listen to my body, then trying to push through the pain and fatigue. I've been trying to be strong, to soldier on, but all my efforts have been for nothing. Denial and desperation rise within me, and I feel the urge to argue against the doctor's statement. But I can't find the words. I sit with tears streaming down my face.

The doctor's gaze weighs on me, but I can't bring myself to meet his eyes. I am trapped in a whirlwind of anger, frustration, and despair. The words keep ringing in my ears.

Unfit for work for the foreseeable future.

The doctor begins to speak once more, but I barely hear him over the din of my thoughts. I nod and murmur responses, but my mind is elsewhere. I can't believe this is now my reality. There is no definitive answer for my recovery.

As I gather my things and stand to leave, the doctor hands me a few leaflets on pain management. I take them without a word and head out of the office. I know I should be grateful for the doctor's concern, but I feel betrayed. My body has let me down in the worst possible way.

The air outside is cold and biting, and I pull my scarf tighter around my face. I flag down a taxi and climb into the back seat. The city streets blur by as the taxi winds through traffic. The neon lights and bustling crowds only add to my feelings of isolation and loneliness. I reach into my bag and pull out my diary. I rustle around for a pen and begin to write.

"I feel like a stranger in my own body. This pain, this illness, it's taken over my life. And no one can see it. It is invisible to the world. I am trapped in my own mind, in my own pain. I don't know how to escape it. I don't know how to get better. All I know is that I am tired. Tired of fighting, tired of struggling. And yet, I can't give up. I can't let this defeat me."

As the taxi pulls up to my house, I close my diary and pay the driver. I step out of the car and walk towards my front door, my mind and heart heavy. Will I ever be able to return to work? Will I ever live a normal life again?

Chapter 9

In It Together

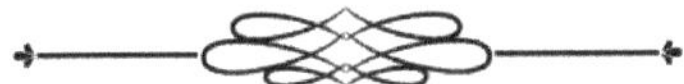

I step into the private hospital, heart pounding with a mixture of anxiety and hope. After five long months of waiting, I'm finally getting a consultation with a top neuro consultant.

My husband walks beside me, and I feel the reassurance of his hand resting gently on my back. We are led to Dr. O'Connor's office, a small, sterile room with a single examination bed on the left and a computer on the desk. The walls are lined with books and medical journals, and the smell of disinfectant is overpowering.

I come prepared with a detailed letter outlining my pain and all the different treatments I've tried, but the consultant doesn't seem interested in it. Instead, he goes straight to taking my history and examining me.

Dr. O'Connor asks me a series of questions, taking notes on his notepad as I speak. I try to remain calm and composed, but my nerves threaten to get the better of me. I am grateful for my husband's presence, as it helps me keep my composure.

"Can you tell me about your pain?" the consultant asks. "When did it start?"

"It started about six months ago. At first, it was just on the right side of my face, but now it's spread to other parts of my body."

"And what triggers the pain?"

"A lot of things. Sometimes brushing my teeth, combing my hair, eating or speaking, and even the wind can cause a jolt of pain."

Dr. O'Connor nods, his face serious as he examines my face and head. "I see sensitivity in your forehead, which isn't consistent with trigeminal neuralgia. It seems like the pain has evolved into something else, but you will have to do more tests before I have a clear picture."

"I already had an MRI," I say, handing him the results. "It didn't show anything."

The consultant glances at the MRI results and hands them back to me. "I recommend further testing, including MRI with contrast, NCS/EMG, and autoimmune tests. We need to rule out other possibilities before we can determine the best course of action."

"That's a lot of tests," I exclaim, my hands trembling with anxiety. My mind races with all the possible outcomes or worse, not finding any answers. The stress and pressure of the appointment triggers something deep inside me that I can't control. Tears begin to stream down my face.

As I try to compose myself, the doctor glares at me in irritation. "I only touched your face with a tissue," he retorts, making me feel even more ashamed and helpless.

I try to explain, "I know, but it's triggered." My words come out in broken sobs. The consultant motions for me to sit on the examination bed, while I struggle to regain my composure.

Despite my efforts to calm down by breathing deeply, I find myself unable to stop crying. The consultant returns to his chair, sitting opposite Anthony who tries to give his two cents. "My wife's pain comes and goes, and stress seems to be a trigger as well."

"We won't know until we try." The way he responds makes it clear my breakdown is an inconvenience. "If nothing helps, we can consider referring you to pain management or consider gamma knife laser treatment. Your case is complex, and I believe a multidisciplinary approach could be beneficial in providing you with the best support to navigate living with chronic pain."

"What is a multidisciplinary approach?" I manage to ask.

"Surrounding yourself with a team of experts who can work together to help you find relief and develop new coping strategies. It's important that you listen to your body and work closely with these professionals to create a plan tailored to your needs."

"I understand." Yet another suggestion to listen to my body, as if I have a choice these days. I am overwhelmed by the thought of having to wait for yet another type of treatment, not to mention scheduling appointments with all these people he is referring to.

"I know it can be frustrating to have to wait, but trust me, this approach can be incredibly effective in helping you find a new normal," he tries to reassure me. "Come back in three months. We should have the results of these tests by then, so we can see how you're doing and make any necessary adjustments to your plan."

"Okay, I'll try to be patient and hope for the best." I bottle up the wave of frustration building in my chest.

"That's the right attitude," Dr. O'Connor says with a smile. "This journey will take time, but with a multidisciplinary approach, you'll have the support you need to get through it."

A knot forms in my stomach at the thought of undergoing more tests and treatments. The consultant's reaction to my meltdown didn't do anything to reassure me that he has my best interests at heart, but I try to reason through it. He's just doing his job. And now I have to do mine. I need to fight for my health.

The appointment ends, leaving me with nothing but more questions and a nagging feeling of disappointment. As my husband and I leave his office, the sterile white hallway stretches before me—a reminder of how far I still have to go.

My husband takes my hand as we step out of the hospital and cross the parking lot. "It's going to be okay." I feel the warmth of his hand, the strength in his voice.

I sigh, tears prickling at the corners of my eyes. "I've been waiting for answers for so long," I whisper, "and now that I finally have a chance to get some, I'm as lost as I was in the beginning. I'm scared."

He pulls me into a hug. "But we're in this together. And no matter what, we'll get through it."

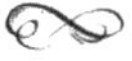

In 2001, I was heading from New Delhi to a conference in Bangalore, a journey of over 2,000 kilometres. On the last leg of the journey, I sat in the back seat of a jeep, waiting for the organizers to tell us which bus to board. Suddenly, a tall, blond man with piercing blue eyes appeared at the window, counting how many of us were inside. His eyes locked onto mine, and I felt a spark.

Needing an excuse to talk to him, I quickly asked the driver, "Could you please let me out? I need to go to the toilet."

The driver nodded, and I approached the blond man. "Excuse me, can you tell me where the restroom is?"

His smile made my heart flutter. "Sure, it's just around the corner. I'll show you."

As we walked, he introduced himself. "I'm Anthony, by the way. I'm helping the organizers."

"I'm Michele," I said, feeling nervous for no reason. "Thank you for your help."

"It's my pleasure," he said warmly. "Are you excited about the conference?"

"Yes, just a bit tired from the trip. It's my first time here."

"No worries," he said. "Bangalore is wonderful, and the conference will be great."

On the first day, we found seats next to each other during the opening session. His presence was comforting, and I felt an immediate sense of ease. He leaned over and whispered a joke about the keynote speaker, making me laugh. His humour was infectious, and I felt myself relaxing more with every passing moment.

We ate all our meals together, sharing stories and discovering common interests. Anthony's enthusiasm for life was contagious. He was surprisingly attentive, ensuring I had everything I needed—from a glass of water during sessions to finding the best spots to grab a quick snack during breaks.

As the sun set on the first day, we found a quiet spot away from the conference hustle. The golden light cast a warm glow around us, and in that moment, Anthony gently pulled me closer. Our first kiss was electric. The connection felt deep, as if we'd known each other forever. I felt an undeniable pull toward him.

For the rest of the conference, we were inseparable. Anthony's caring nature shone through in small gestures. He remembered my favourite drink and surprised me with it during a particularly long session. When I expressed an interest in a particular topic, he introduced me to speakers and attendees who shared my passion, helping me make valuable connections.

People around us noticed our closeness, amazed when I would tell them we just met. Anthony's humour and attentiveness quickly wove a deep connection between us. It became clear from the start: it was love at first sight.

I was 18, and Anthony was two years older than me. By the end of the conference, his thoughtfulness, kindness, and love created a bond that felt like it had been a lifetime in the making. He was everything I'd been dreaming of in a man—caring, loving, and a true gentleman.

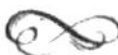

Twenty years have passed. We are still inseparable, having weathered various storms and challenges during our dating years and our marriage. But we have never faced anything like this.

I lean back against the passenger seat, replaying the appointment in my mind. The consultant was efficient, but I'd waited five months for this appointment only to be told I need more tests and more appointments. I mentally run through all the questions I had written down before the appointment. He hadn't asked me if I had any questions. I had placed so much hope on this one meeting. And now I'm back where I started.

The drive back to Limerick from Dublin will be just as long and painful as the drive here a total of five hours for a consultation that didn't even last 20 minutes.

I gaze out the window, somewhat refreshed by the landscape unfurling before me. Along the highway, cattle and sheep graze peacefully amidst rolling hills and lush greenery. The tranquil scenery calms my racing thoughts, even if just for a moment.

I can't give up. I won't give up.

I have to keep fighting for my health and for answers. And I know that my husband will be by my side, every step of the way.

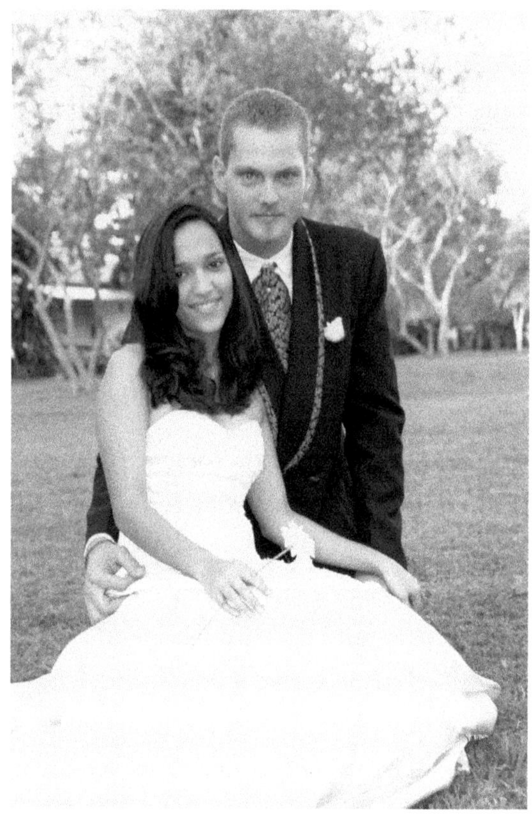

Rio de Janeiro - RJ - Brazil

Chapter 10

Opening Pandora's Box

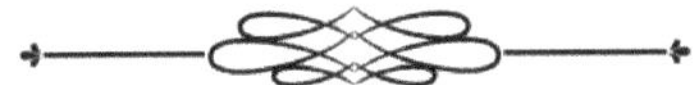

The afternoon sun streams into the room as I attempt to focus on the details around me. My therapist suggested mindful practices such as this to help escape the constant ache. The room I share with my husband is simple but cosy, with magnolia walls and wood skirting boards. Our bed is the focal point, where I am tucked in beneath a soft white quilt and plush pillows. A nightstand beside me holds a lamp and a few books stacked neatly.

Across from the bed is a bay window, cracked open, letting in a gentle breeze. The room is a safe place I can hide from the world. I close my eyes and let the warmth from the sunshine soothe my aching body.

But as I lie here, worries start to press down on me. After nine months, I'm still waiting for insurance to cover my loss of income "in case of illness." I applied as soon as my health began to decline and went through the right channels, but they haven't responded yet. I even asked my family solicitor to write them, twice. But still, nothing. I feel like they don't care about my situation, like they don't understand the stress and anxiety this waiting is causing me.

Every day, I worry about our dwindling finances. And it's my fault. If only this neuralgia would disappear, I could get back to work and help support my family. I close my eyes and try to push away the thoughts of financial strain. But the fears continue to nag at me.

Why can't I just get back to my normal self? I know I should be grateful for moments like this, when the pain subsides for a few minutes, but I only feel anger and resentment towards this illness that has taken over my life.

My phone rings. The caller ID shows me it's Peter, my financial advisor. I take a deep breath to steady my nerves.

"Hello?"

"Hi, Michele. How are you today?"

"I'm okay, just trying to keep my head above water."

"I understand," Peter says. "I wanted to check in and see if you've heard from the insurance company yet."

"Nothing. It's been radio silence." I feel a knot form in my stomach. "What's going on? Why hasn't the paperwork been processed yet?"

"I'm not sure, but I'll follow up with them. In the meantime, let's focus on finding other ways to make ends meet."

Peter means well, but his words add to my inner turmoil. I am a prisoner in my own body, unable to escape either the pain or the financial struggles that surround me.

"I appreciate your help, Peter," I say, my voice breaking. "I just want to get back to my normal self and help provide for my family."

"I understand, and we'll get there," Peter reassures me. "In the meantime, try to focus on taking care of yourself and your health. Everything else will fall into place."

I hang up the phone, feeling a mixture of frustration and gratitude. I know Peter is doing everything he can to help, but it's still a difficult situation to be in. I take a deep breath, close my eyes, and whisper a prayer for strength and guidance.

"Lord, please make a way."

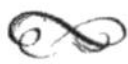

As I walk into the primary care centre, I feel the usual sense of trepidation. The waiting room is empty, save for metal chairs with blue fabric seats that line the wall. I hear a child screaming from the room to my right, the cries echoing through sterile halls. It mirrors the chaos and pain I have been living with for months. Too bad I'm an adult. It might be weird if I start screaming to express how I'm feeling. I sit down, trying to calm my racing heart and steady my breathing.

I've visited countless doctors and specialists, but no one seems to be able to do anything about my chronic pain. I'm tired of taking prescription medications and going through endless tests and scans, only to be told nothing can be done to help me. The financial stress of paying for all these appointments and scans is taking its toll. If there was an end in sight, I would be able to focus on that, but this road is going on forever.

I close my eyes, trying to focus on the present moment and let my thoughts drift away. I hear my name and open my eyes again. A woman with a British accent stands before me.

"My name is Paula. Please follow me."

I follow her through a maze of winding hallways, their walls plastered with informational posters and leaflets. We climb a flight of stairs and stop in front of five doors, each one leading to a different type of therapist. Paula opens the door to her small office and gestures for me to take a seat. The room is cramped, with a small child's desk in the corner and filing cabinets lining the walls. There are two chairs, and I choose a brown one that looks comfortable.

"Welcome, Michele," Paula says, sitting across from me. "Your GP has referred you to us, and I will be going through some paperwork before we get started. Is that okay with you?"

I nod, apprehensive. This is a new therapist, a new location, and almost a year into my chronic pain

"Why is it that you're seeking help from our service?" Paula asks, pen in hand.

I begin to explain what has happened over the past several months, but it feels like my words are coming out in a jumbled rush. Tears well up in my eyes.

"Okay, let's scale it back a bit, Michele. Can you take a few deep breaths?" Paula's tone is warm, and I follow her advice. I can feel my heart rate slowing and the tightness in my chest easing as I breathe deeply. "Let's start again, shall we?"

I try to put into words the constant pain, frustration, and exhaustion I've been feeling since this ordeal began.

"It's been a rough few months," I say, my voice barely above a whisper. "I've been to countless doctors, specialists, and therapists, but no one seems to be able to help me. I feel like I'm just being passed from one person to the next, and no one is actually listening to me. The financial stress of all these appointments is overwhelming, and I'm scared of what the future holds."

Paula nods. "I know this is a difficult journey for you," she says. "But I want you to know that we're going to work together to help you cope with your physical pain and the emotional turmoil that comes with it."

"Thank you," I murmur.

"Can you tell me more about your journey so far, Michele?" she prompts.

I begin once more to share my story, starting at the beginning. I tell her about the ongoing tests and appointments, the chronic pain that never seems to go away, the frustration of not being able to work or live a normal life. I tell her about the financial stress, the weight of uncertainty, and the constant exhaustion.

Paula nods and remains focused, making me feel heard.

"Michele, has anything traumatic happened in your life? Have you ever experienced any abuse?"

My body tenses. The words I know I need to say feel like jagged stones in my mouth. I take a deep breath, trying to steady my racing heart. "Um ... I was abused as a child," I confess, feeling shame weigh heavily on my chest, making it hard to breathe.

Five years ago, I briefly mentioned this to another therapist, but as soon as I said the word "abuse," I froze up and couldn't say anything else about it. I changed the subject ... yet here, with Paula, this truth about my past is finally being given a chance to emerge. It's not easy but I know I have to be willing to do whatever it takes to get better, even if it means rummaging through dark parts of me that have been kept in the shadows.

"It's not your fault, Michele," she says softly. "Whatever happened to you was not your fault."

Her words feel like a balm to my soul. I let out a shaky sigh and tears fill my eyes. At the same time, a little bit of the burden lifts from my shoulders.

"There are support groups and therapy programmes designed specifically for survivors of childhood abuse," Paula tells me. "I highly recommend that you look into them, Michele. It could be a valuable step in your healing journey."

"Thank you," I say, although I don't think I'm ready for something like that yet.

"What's the main thing that's hard for you right now?" she prods.

I hesitate, trying to find the words to express what I'm feeling. "I'm trying to control everything, but there is nothing in my life I can actually control right now!"

Paula nods, "That's common for survivors of trauma. But right now, you need to learn to let go. It will help you see the patterns holding you back so your health can begin to improve."

"Let go?" I repeat. The idea feels foreign.

"Yes." Paula's voice is firm but kind. "It can be a scary thought, but it's necessary for your healing. You've been holding on to so much pain and hurt for so long. It's time to start letting it go, little by little."

I look around the therapy room for anything that can take my attention away from what Paula has just said. I'm suddenly overwhelmed with emotions, and I take another deep, shaky breath.

"Michele, you're doing great. Just take it one step at a time. This is a journey, and it will take time, but you are not alone. Remember that." She brings the session to a close.

I gather my things and make my way back through the halls and down the stairs. As I step outside and head toward the parking area, the warmth of the sun on my skin doesn't ease the turmoil inside me. My mind is a whirlpool of conflicting thoughts and emotions. Is it possible to ever truly heal from my past?

The idea of letting go, of giving up the only sense of control I've ever known, is overwhelming. Mentioning my childhood abuse feels like I've just opened Pandora's box, exposing a part of me I had kept locked away for so long. How am I supposed to just let go when holding it carefully inside helped me survive?

I sit behind the steering wheel, trying to make sense of all that was shared in the office. Guilt, shame, anger, loss of control—they all swim through my mind. I take another deep breath, trying to ground myself, but the tears begin to fall. Once they start, it is as though the floodgates have opened. They keep pouring out.

Chapter 11

Waiting Game

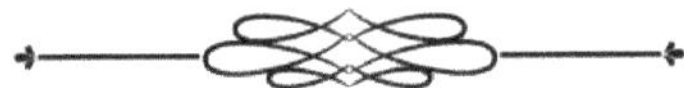

My husband and I drive to Dublin for a follow up visit with Dr. O'Connor. I'm nervous about meeting the consultant again. Last time, I lost control of my emotions in part because of the man's hasty manner.

We arrive early and Anthony steers into a free parking space in the underground car park. It's cold, and the car park isn't heated. We step into the frigid air. In my mind, I'm trying to play out how the meeting is going to go.

"Honey, please try to control your emotions this time," my husband says. "It will be hard for him to assess you if you break out in tears again."

"I can't promise that, Anthony. It depends if I get a burst of pain at the time or not, but I will try." I hold firmly to my pink folder, which contains my records from St. Vincent's Hospital, copies of my two recent brain MRIs, and records of blood tests I obtained from my own doctor.

We take the elevator to the fourth floor and find the designated door. I walk in and notify the receptionist that I'm here to see the consultant neurologist. He is with a patient, so I sit down and look around the waiting area. There are only three of us: an elderly couple and another man whose movements are halting and shaky. I wonder if he has Parkinson's.

The elderly woman has a bright smile on her face. She asks me if I've read the doctor's book, and I tell her I haven't.

"Well, I haven't read much of it, but I like it so far," she says. "I am going to have him sign it for me today." For a split second, I imagine myself as that elderly lady, but I quickly dismiss the thought. Instead, I marvel at her bravery, positivity, and warmth. She doesn't know me from Adam, yet she makes small talk, which eases my nervousness.

Dr. O'Connor exits his office and beckons the couple. The woman struggles to stand up, and her husband lends a hand. As soon as she's on her feet, she strikes up a conversation with the doctor. "Your book is very impressive," she remarks to him. Dr. O'Connor beams and thanks her. A moment later, he guides them down the hallway to his consulting room.

My mind swims with questions as they go in for the consultation. What's the source of my pain? Can I get rid of it? Will my body recover naturally? After almost a year of searching, I'm still at a loss for answers. When will the insurance company pay out? I'm spending money without any assurance of answers.

After about ten minutes, the woman reemerges from the consulting room, disrupting my thoughts. The woman stops in front of me.

"I got him to sign it," she announces with conviction. "He's a great doctor. Don't worry. You're in good hands." She walks towards the door. Anthony opens it for them while the elderly man helps his wife keep her balance. Their footsteps fade away, leaving me with a glimmer of hope.

Dr. O'Connor emerges from his office and calls my name. I stand up, take a deep breath, and follow him into the consultation room. He goes over my last report, going through the MRI and the nerve conductor studies on my hand.

"You don't have carpal tunnel, but I guess you already know that."

I nod, waiting for him to continue.

"You don't have an aneurysm in your brain, and you don't have MS, so you won't be needing a wheelchair. As far as we can see, there is no tumour in your brain either. So that is all positive." He looks at me and smiles. "As far as I am concerned, you are not going to die any time soon, and that is great news."

"But that doesn't explain my pain," I say. "It doesn't explain why my face is half numb. It doesn't explain why I am so fatigued." I'm not worried about tumours and aneurysms. I want a fix for this constant, invisible pain.

"I am sorry, but I don't have all the answers," Dr. O'Connor replies. "Your body will settle in its own time, and no one knows how much time that might take. Each person is different. You will need to be patient as we find out what works for you." He repeats the need for a multidisciplinary approach, just as he did last time. "Going to a psychologist will also help, as well as other types of therapists to see what makes a difference."

I feel deflated again. Dr. O'Connor can probably see I am holding back tears. I wonder why I bothered to drive all the way up here, pay for fuel, parking, and the consultation to hear him tell me what I already knew. The same thing he told me last time.

"Look, it's very difficult for me to come all the way here. It's also expensive. I am on a waiting list with Dr. Ryan in Limerick. Could you please at least send a letter referring me to him? It might help expedite the situation."

He agrees, adding, "I know him well. He is a very good doctor,"

I thank him and get my bag and pink folder from the floor. At least the entire trip wasn't a waste if I get this referral. I look back at him and ask, "Have you seen people with a similar condition to mine?"

"Yes," he replies, "it sorts itself out. You will see, but just remember, it takes time. But you should be happy to know you will not end up in a wheelchair. You are young, with your life ahead of you. Try this new medication I am prescribing and keep positive. You will get there."

On the way back to the car, my face starts throbbing and the crying that I held back inside the office comes in full force. I keep my eyes glued to the floor in the elevator as tears begin to fall.

I continue to cry when we reach the car. Anthony tries to reassure me, telling me to look at the bright side—I won't die or be in a wheelchair anytime soon.

Great! I am alive—but how do I live with something that no one else can see? How can I strive to get better when I don't know what the root cause is? I can call it whatever it is—facial neuralgia, or whatever—but the reality is that it's controlling me. Each and every day, each and every minute.

I don't know how strong I am or will have to be to get on with this ... for how long?

I let out a scream, pounding my fist against the car door. "Nine months! I can't believe it's been nine months of this!" My voice trembles with rage and tears. "Relentless pain, countless medications, useless treatments, and still no answers!"

My breathing is ragged, and I can feel the heat of my fury burning through me. "I'm so tired of this! How can they just brush me off like this? Do they think it's all in my head?" I slam my fist again, the dull thud echoing my frustration. "I'm fed up with hearing people say I look fine. THEY HAVE NO IDEA WHAT I'M GOING THROUGH!"

I collapse back into the seat, exhausted from the outburst, tears streaming down my face. My husband reaches over, squeezing my hand gently. "I'm sorry, Honey. We will keep looking for answers. Maybe Dr. Ryan will have more insights," he says softly, but the uncertainty in his voice mirrors my own doubts.

I let out a bitter laugh. "I'm still on the urgent waiting list to see him, Anthony. It's been nine months since I was referred, and I still haven't heard back. That's why we went private to Dr. O'Connor, and still we had to wait five months for that first appointment."

He sighs. "I know, I know. But we can't give up. Maybe we should try some of the other therapies our friends suggested. The chiropractor in Cork, perhaps?"

I shake my head, feeling the weight of the unending pain and emotional exhaustion. "Can we just stop talking about it? Please, Anthony. Just ... play some classical music instead."

He nods and reaches for the radio, tuning it to a classical station, RTE Lyric. The soothing notes fill the car, but they do little to calm the storm inside me. I stare out the window, watching the countryside pass by, blurred by my tears. The constant pain gnaws at my body, and the lack of answers feels like a weight crushing my spirit.

Outwardly, I may look fine, but inside, I'm a wreck. My mental strength is crumbling, and all the positive thoughts I've tried to hold onto are slipping away.

As we continue our journey from Dublin to Limerick, I close my eyes and let the music wash over me, trying to find some semblance of peace amidst the chaos. I feel awful for venting. I need to be strong—for myself, for my husband, and for my children. My face is on fire, and the crying hasn't helped. My head is hurting even worse.

The frustration and despair linger, a reminder of the battle I fight every single day.

I lie on an ultrasound bed, inner tension rapidly building. The technician is focusing on my thyroid, ignoring my requests to examine my neck and face.

"Excuse me, but can you please check a few inches up on my neck and face?" I ask again, trying to keep the impatience from creeping into my voice.

"I'm sorry, but I can only follow the referral letter," the technician replies, not even making eye contact.

I sigh heavily. Is no one going to take my concerns seriously?

"Listen, I've been experiencing numbness and fullness in my neck and face, as well as shooting and stabbing pain. Can't you just take a quick look while you're already here?" I plead.

The technician's expression remains an emotionless mask. "I'm sorry, but I can only follow the guidelines provided in the referral letter. You'll need to wait for another appointment and referral to have that area examined."

His dismissive attitude only fuels the frustration simmering within me. Time and again, it feels like my pain and concerns are being ignored, like I am just another number in the medical system.

"Can you at least tell me what kind of cyst it is? Could it be causing the numbness in my face?" I ask, desperate.

The technician hesitates for a moment. "The cyst on your thyroid is fluid-filled, so there's nothing to worry about," he says, sounding almost relieved to be done with the appointment, done with this emotional, needy patient.

As I return to the waiting area, disappointment wraps around me like a suffocating blanket. The medical system is a labyrinth, and I am lost in its maze. The technician's uninterested attitude only adds insult to injury. Eleven months of chronic pain, countless doctors and specialists, and still no answers.

I remind myself that I should be grateful for the good news about the cyst that was first detected on my MRI, but it feels like a small victory in the grand scheme of things. I try to ground myself with deep breathing, yet the pain in my face and neck intensifies with each intake of breath. It feels like I'm losing control, not just of my body, but of my mind and emotions as well.

I pick up my journal and begin to write, trying to make sense of the jumbled thoughts in my head. As I write, I realise that perhaps my husband is right. Maybe my mind is causing me to feel even more fatigued and exhausted due to all the information I am consuming. Media, podcasts, books on my current condition, and self-help techniques, not to mention all the geopolitical events going on. But how can I control that? How can I stop myself from constantly thinking and questioning and worrying?

I need to find a way to heal not only my physical pain, but my emotional and mental pain as well. In my journal, I jot down a note to discuss this with Paula in our next therapy session.

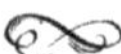

A new year has begun. It is January 2020, and I still have no answers. After six months of anticipation, I brace against the chilly air to make my way to University Hospital Limerick for my long-awaited appointment with Dr. Ryan.

The hospital atmosphere is starkly different from the private facility in Dublin. The corridors, adorned with white and blue metal chairs, are a sea of people in every nook and cranny. The outpatient ward on the ground floor is a hub of activity. The secretary's corner desk is surrounded by files, both neatly stacked and sprawled out haphazardly. All chairs are occupied, at least 20 people seated, with more standing in the corridor.

As I hand my appointment letter to the secretary, I express my hope to see the main consultant, instead of a junior doctor, since I have waited for so long.

"I will see what we can do for you." She makes a note on my chart.

"Dr. Ryan's clinic is a busy place, isn't it?" I ask, stating the obvious.

"Yes, but this area is also for other consultants and doctors." She instructs me to find a chair and wait for the nurse.

In the corridor, just beyond the main hall, doors line both sides, each leading to different doctors and consultants. Anthony, seeming to sense my apprehension, stands by my side as there is no place for him to sit. I clutch my pink folder.

"Michele Roys." The nurse calls my name, chart in hand. I stand up. She ushers me to a room five doors down the long corridor. "Sit here, and we'll take your weight and measurements." The nurse points me to a chair. "You're 56.5 kg," she reports, writing it on my chart. The number hits me hard.

Growing up in Brazil, I was surrounded by explicit music, dancing, and the constant pressure to fit in. At 15 years old, I was willing to do anything to be part of the crowd, to be accepted and liked.

My best friend, two years older than me, was tall, pretty, and wore lots of earrings. She was the essence of cool, so I took everything she told me to heart. We flipped through different magazines—health magazines, exercise guides, and pages filled with gorgeous models.

"Shelly, you've got to be thin. The clothes have to be skimpy. That's what the guys like," she told me one day.

I'd always been slender, but even the slightest bit of tummy bothered me. I was only 46 kilos, but also fairly short at 1.52 meters. I wanted the boys to like me, so I started rollerblading and skating, hanging out with a lot of boys, wearing baggy pants and tight, short tops. And it worked. I enjoyed being the centre of attention. I had a lot of friends, but I wanted more.

One day, I read a magazine article about a girl who ate whatever she wanted and then just puked it up. It sounded disgusting. Yet there I was, having to count my calories and watch everything I ate to keep my body in shape. I was athletic and joined in every single soccer game, volleyball match, rollerblading event—anything that came around. But that thought lingered in my mind—throwing up to stay thin.

I asked my friend, who was from Argentina and knew about all sorts of things.

"Yes, I've been doing that for a while now. I haven't put on any weight," she told me.

I decided it wouldn't hurt to try.

And so, it began. Once a day, I would eat a big meal—either lunch or dinner, depending on how my day was going. After a few minutes, I would visit the bathroom and kneel on the cold, brown tiles in front of the toilet bowl. I would hold my hair back with one hand while steadying myself against the wall with the other. My stomach would clench as I forced myself to throw up everything I'd just eaten.

Part of me felt relieved, thinking that my body took what it needed in those few minutes the food was in my stomach. I convinced myself it was just fat I was getting rid of—unnecessary, unwanted.

But deep down, it fed the feeling that I was not good enough. I had to work hard to make myself liked and accepted, even if it meant doing this. Even if it meant hurting myself.

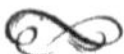

I was 52 kg three months ago. Before this health crisis, I was at a steady 50 kg. It's not like I've been overindulging in my dark chocolate cravings, but the medications have taken their toll. I continue to gain weight.

The nurse takes my blood pressure, inquiring about my current medications; she jots down the vitals. "Wait outside. I'll make sure the main consultant gets your chart."

I head back outside, sharing my dismay with Anthony. "Can you believe it? I'm 56.5 kilos. I'm gutted."

"Honey, your health has changed, and it's winter," Anthony reassures me. "A little extra weight is good for warmth." His comforting smile and the squeeze of his hand ease my frustration, if only momentarily.

Despite Anthony's reassurance, my weight is yet another thing no longer under my control. The side effects of medication have left me feeling bloated and uncomfortable. I despise them so much that I pleaded with my doctor to discontinue them. They not only fail to alleviate my pain but also make me groggy, unwell, and nauseous.

Thirty minutes later, my name is called, and we follow Dr. Ryan down the corridor. Annoyance over my weight lingers, but I focus on the impending consultation. Expecting a brief meeting, I provide a concise summary, hoping for more time for his questions and examination.

"Mrs. Roys, your case is quite intriguing," Dr. Ryan remarks, delving into my history, pain levels, and sensations, as well as the medications and treatments I've tried since the onset of my condition. I appreciate the attention, and he conducts a thorough examination. The fullness, numbness, and crawling sensation on the right side of my face are not typical trigeminal neuralgia, he explains. Instead, it appears to be an atypical TN, possibly bilateral.

"Let's take a closer look at your MRI images," he suggests, emphasising the importance of a multidisciplinary approach in dealing with complex facial neuralgia cases. He encourages me to maintain hope. Unlike the consultations with Dr. O'Connor that barely lasted 20 minutes, this one extends well over 40 minutes. I am grateful for the thorough examination.

A few weeks later, a letter from Dr. Ryan arrives. Despite inconclusive MRI images, he diagnoses my condition as facial neuralgia and trigeminal autonomic cephalgia on the right side of my face. The revelation explains the tears in my right eye during flare-ups.

He suggests trying another medication for three months before my next review. This diagnosis gives me a renewed sense of hope, even though I wish my condition could be seen on an image to substantiate my pain. Friends still tell me, "You look just fine," and I want proof that this isn't all in my head.

Chapter 12

When the World Stopped

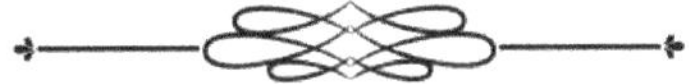

The day the lockdown measures are announced, it feels like the ground beneath me has shifted, leaving me unmoored. The pandemic has brought the world to a standstill, and with it, my own life unravels. My husband is unable to work due to the restrictions, adding additional financial strain to our already fragile situation.

The boys' schooling becomes a chaotic endeavour. My youngest, who's studying at an all-Irish school, is inundated with Gaelic assignments—a language I don't speak. Each morning, I'm greeted by pages of incomprehensible text and instructions that seem like they're from another world.

"Mom, I don't understand any of this," he says, defeat in his voice as he holds an open book in front of me.

I look at the page, feeling utterly defeated. "I'm sorry, sweetheart. I wish I could help. Let's try to use a translator and see if that helps," I suggest, though my own panic is barely masked. We stumble through the assignments, trying to piece together the meaning with the help of an online translator, but the process is slow.

Meanwhile, my eldest is struggling with the stress of moving from 2nd year to 3rd year, a crucial time with junior certificate exams looming on the horizon. His academic stress is compounded by the turbulence of teenage years and the restrictive lockdown measures. The walls of our home seem to close in on him, and his frustration becomes more palpable with each passing day.

"This is so unfair!" he yells one evening, slamming his book down with a force that makes the table shake. "I can't focus with everything going on. And why can't I see my friends? I hate this!"

I try to offer comfort, but my own patience is stretched thin. "I know it's tough. We're all struggling. Just do your best, okay?"

I am also suffering the weight of exhaustion with this unbearable condition. My medication leaves me drowsy and irritable, like a thick fog settling over my mind. My husband takes care of daily chores while I try to help my boys with their schoolwork, but the constant pain and brain fog make it nearly impossible to focus.

I call my boys to bring their laptops to my room, where I attempt to assist them with their scholastic needs.

"Mom, can you check this for me?" my youngest asks, carrying his laptop to my bedside.

I look at the screen, but the words swim in and out of focus. "I ... I'm sorry, I'm having a hard time concentrating. Maybe try looking it up online?" I feel utterly useless, my attempts to focus on their work failing as the pain and fatigue overwhelm me.

As I close my eyes and try to breathe deeply, the soothing strains of classical music from the radio offer a brief respite. Even in these moments of calm, the weight of the pandemic's impact on my life and my family's well-being remains ever-present. Each day is a battle to find a sliver of normalcy amid the chaos; small victories feel overshadowed by the immense challenges we face.

In this new reality, the blend of chronic pain, emotional strain, and the constant pressure of an uncertain future is almost too much to bear. The comfort of our old routines has been replaced by a cycle of anxiety and frustration amplified by the isolation of lockdown.

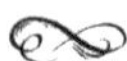

I sit on my trusty brown couch, facing the sun-drenched bay window in my bedroom. Despite the warmth and comfort the sun brings, I feel a sense of disconnection, made even more pronounced by the fact that my therapy sessions with my new therapist, Anne, are now conducted online due to the pandemic. The physical distance between us only amplifies the emotional distance I feel.

"I don't know why I find it so hard to rest," I admit to Anne. "I just feel like I need to keep moving, like being still makes me useless." I grasp my grey fluffy rabbit keychain for comfort.

Anne nods. "Interesting. Let's dive into that a little more."

I hesitate. The thought of exploring these emotions terrifies me.

Anne must sense my hesitation. "Why don't you try to name what it is you fear," she suggests.

"My fear is that if I ever stop completely, I will sink into a deep depression," I try to explain. "I don't know what that feels like, but I do know that I have to keep busy to avoid dealing with these emotions that keep surfacing and the critical voices inside me that never stop." My body feels weighted down with lead, and every movement is a struggle against the pain that grips me.

"You're making progress, Michele," Anne reassures me, her voice soft and soothing. "Can you tell me about the different inner voices that criticise you?" she asks.

I take a deep breath and try to put into words the internal battle I've been facing. "There's the taskmaster, who constantly reminds me of all the things I haven't accomplished each day. The judge, who holds me to impossibly high standards. And the sergeant general, who combines all three of these voices. In the background, there's a calm and wise part of me, but it's often drowned out by the critical voices."

"That's quite a battle you're fighting within yourself, isn't it, Michele?"

I nod silently.

"How does that feel for you? Can you describe it?"

"It feels like a storm that never ends," I whisper, my voice trembling with the force of the emotions I'm trying to express. "I am struggling to find my footing in this dark, uncharted territory. It's been a gruelling 20 months, and it feels like my inner selves are at war."

"Can we stay here for a moment longer, Michele?" my therapist asks. "I don't want you to miss this opportunity. Are there any other parts of you that need to be heard?"

I close my eyes, take a deep breath, and allow my thoughts to flow freely. The physical pain I have been suppressing, trying my best to ignore, suddenly takes centre stage.

"I try to pretend it's not there," I explain, warm tears stealing down my face. "I try to make others believe that all is well, but the truth is, the pain is constant, and sometimes it spikes to unbearable levels. I am afraid to acknowledge it because I fear it will consume me. I don't want to surrender, accepting this as my fate. But what if that's exactly what I need to do?"

I sob, feeling as if my innermost world has just been exposed. I have been denying this illness even though it has kept me from doing everything I was once used to doing.

"Let's talk a bit more about your fear, Michele," my therapist suggests. "What do you fear most about acknowledging your pain and surrendering to it?"

I take a moment to gather my thoughts. "I fear losing control. I fear losing the drive that has pushed me to succeed, to be the best I can be. If I give in to my pain, I'm afraid I will become a shadow of the person I want to be, that I'll be unable to accomplish anything or make a difference in the world. I fear losing the fire that has burned within me for so long."

"That's a lot of fear, Michele." My therapist nods, her expression one of compassion. "But I want you to understand that recognizing your pain, giving it a voice, is not giving in to it. It's not about surrendering; it's about taking charge. You are taking charge of your own healing journey and finding a way to live a meaningful life despite your physical pain."

Her words resonate deeply. "I get it. It's about finding a balance—a way to rest, heal, and still be motivated to reach my goals, even if it's in a different way than I used to."

"Exactly," she agrees. "It's about honouring both your pain and your ambition while finding a way to live a life full of meaning. It's about taking the time to heal, to recharge, and then gathering the courage to stand back up and keep pushing forward."

I can feel weight lifting from my shoulders as I realise that acknowledging my pain is not a failure. Instead, it can be a way to discover a new path forward.

Perhaps this path will lead me to a life of balance, joy, and fulfilment in measures I have never known before.

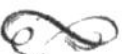

My life has been a whirlwind of pain and chaos for the past two years. It's like I'm treading water in a stormy sea, struggling to keep my head above the crashing waves. My days are filled with trying to manage my own physical pain, deal with my boys' hormonal outbursts, and keep up with my siblings' never-ending drama. The pain is relentless, and it's starting to control more and more of my life.

I've always been someone who throws themselves into being busy, using it as a shield to protect myself from confronting what's going on inside—secrets that have haunted me for years. But it seems that my busyness has only been a way to deceive myself. My therapist called me out on it by pointing out that I always bring up other things during our sessions instead of dealing with the real pain lurking inside.

I know I need to confront the hurt and trauma from my childhood, the emotional turmoil and shame I've been carrying. But the fear of what others will say, what they will think when they look at me is paralyzing. I'm not ready to confront these issues head-on.

The secrets I've kept hidden for so long are eating away at me. I feel cracks appearing, and I've been frantically patching them up, trying to hold myself together, but it's becoming increasingly hard to keep everything in check.

The constant physical pain makes it hard to focus, and I'm running out of professionals to turn to for answers. The thought of opening up to myself and risking the emotions flooding out like a bursting dam terrifies me.

But I have to do it. I must face the hard work of self-reflection and understand the decisions I've made, no matter how painful they may be. I long for healing and relief. Maybe there's a light at the end of the tunnel, but I need to walk through the darkness to get there.

As I sit reflecting on the conversation with my therapist, my thoughts drift to the past, the journey that brought me to this point. Growing up in Brazil, I was exposed to poverty, violence, and abuse at a young age.

In my early teen years, a chasm developed that separated me from my family. The words from scripture that often echoed in my mind were, "When my father or mother abandon me, the Lord will lift me up." But it was not my parents who had abandoned me. It was I who had fled, unable to bear the burden of a secret I had kept since I was eight.

One Sunday morning when I was about 12, my mother was visiting my ailing aunty. My sisters and I were home alone with our stepfather. My younger sister ran into our room, her face ghostly pale, to tell my older sister and me what had just happened to her. Our stepfather, while drunk, asked my little sister to massage his penis while he watched a 'Formula One' race on TV.

We fled the house and took refuge with a neighbour for the day, waiting for my mother to return. When mom arrived, I sat in the neighbour's kitchen, barely speaking, consumed by feelings of guilt and anger towards myself. As the sun set, I realised this might be the only opportunity I had to speak the truth and prevent further harm to my sisters.

I started to sob uncontrollably. My mother and the kind neighbour tried to calm me down and assuage my fears that nothing had happened to my sister. She had run to get help, and we were all safe. But the knot in my throat grew tighter as I struggled between revealing the truth and keeping it hidden.

One choice might mean sending my stepfather to jail and breaking our family apart. The other choice would result in damaging those I cared for, especially my younger siblings.

Finally, I blurted out, "It happened to me, too. What he just tried with her, and more. It's been going on since I was eight!" My tears, anger, and years of pent-up emotions erupted all at once. I rocked back and forth, hitting myself against the wall as I clung to my knees.

My mother rushed to comfort me, but the hurt was too deep. My family would be torn apart because of me. I felt like I had shattered their lives into a million pieces, and there was no way to fix it. Betraying my stepfather's trust and breaking apart my family became a weight I would carry with me forever.

My grandma came to visit us and quickly made plans to get us out of that situation. I don't know how much she knew or who else my mother told. All I remember is moving away from our stepfather and feeling guilty for everything.

The memories of that day are mostly blocked from my mind, but I can still see myself sitting in that corner, on the cold floor, my back against the wall, sobbing and scratching myself.

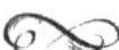

With my mom sick and my stepfather gone, the five of us kids were often left to fend for ourselves. I didn't know if Mom was actually sick or overwhelmed with frustration and anger about everything that happened. I would often see her crying, for hours on end it seemed. I felt responsible.

After my grandma came to take us from Goiania, we moved to her place in Ceilandia, Brasilia, for a little while. Once she managed to arrange a place, we settled into a small house at the end of a bigger two-story home owned by a landlady with three kids. It was a shed she'd converted into a living space. The walls were bright yellow, with a tiny kitchen, an outside bathroom, and one bedroom with a single bed and a mattress on the floor for Mom and the five of us kids.

One day, I answered a knock at the door. It was the landlady. "The rent is due for this week," she said. "Your parents haven't paid last week's rent either. Can you ask them when they'll be paying? Otherwise, I'll have to ask you all to leave."

My oldest sister Clara, who stood at the door with me, tried to explain. "Our parents are separated, and Mom is sick. We'll try to pay. Can you give us another week?" The landlady looked at us, bewilderment on her face, but reluctantly agreed.

After she left, I asked Clara, "What are we going to do? We'll end up on the streets if we can't pay the rent."

"God has to do a miracle for us," she answered simply.

I turned to my youngest sister, Mariane, who was nine, and asked her to watch our two younger brothers while Clara and I went out to find a way to pay the rent. We searched the house and found a Christian reflection written on a single sheet of paper. We put on our nicest clothes and walked down the dirt road toward the main town. Being small, we squeezed under the metal bars on the bus to avoid paying the fare.

By the bus stop was a newsstand run by a lady. We approached her nervously.

"Excuse me, Ma'am," Clara asked, "we were wondering if you could help us with something."

The lady, with her black hair pulled back in a ponytail, looked up from her work. "What do you need, girls?"

"We have this reflection," Clara explained, holding out the paper. "Our mother is sick, and our father is no longer with us. We need to help pay the rent and buy food for our brothers and sisters. Could you possibly photocopy this for us? We can't afford to pay for it, but it would really help us out."

The lady's face softened. "You poor things. How many copies do you need?"

"As many as you can spare," I answered, hoping for at least a few.

She nodded. "I'll give you 20 copies. Will that be enough?"

We could hardly believe our luck. "Thank you so much!" Clara and I answered in unison. She went into the back, and we heard the hum of the photocopier.

When she returned, she handed us the copies with a gentle smile. "I hope this helps."

"It does, more than you know," Clara replied, her voice trembling a bit. "Thank you."

From there, we went from shop to shop, asking to speak to the managers or owners. Here we were, 12 and 13 years old, knocking on doors to get the money we needed for rent. Amazingly, we found some very nice people along the way who donated money in exchange for the reflection.

At the end of the day, we headed to the supermarket to buy a loaf of bread, a bottle of milk, a six-pack of yogurt—a special treat for the kids—and some eggs. We had just enough money left over to pay part of the rent, so we brought it to the landlady, happy to be fulfilling our promise.

This became our life for the next few months—we couldn't afford to go to school because we had to provide for our family, and it was all my fault.

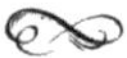

At thirteen, I decided to leave my mother and siblings behind and move in with family friends. My brothers' tear-stained faces haunted me as they cried themselves to sleep each night, sometimes calling out for our absent stepfather. Their pain weighed heavily on me, yet I couldn't bring myself to reveal the truth behind our stepfather's departure.

Guilt and sorrow consumed me over the next four years, leaving me with no choice but to flee as far as I could, seeking solace in the distant lands of India. Although my connection with my siblings was never completely severed, I always felt ashamed at how much they struggled growing up.

What does my current physical pain have to do with my past? The answer eludes me, but the tension that creeps into my face and the knot in my throat leaves me with no doubt—there is a connection.

I was just a child then, innocent and unaware. I did what I could to protect myself. Perhaps it's time to heal. Time to break free from denial and accept what happened. Time to let go of the guilt I have carried for thirty long years.

But is healing truly available for someone like me?

I want to cling to the promises of compassion and forgiveness that my faith tells me is there for me, but although part of me believes it, another part tells me I still have to work hard to prove myself worthy. It feels impossible to simply surrender to the compassion and love that Jesus has for me. How can I start to show the same kindness to myself that He has shown me through His presence remaining through the most difficult moments of my life?

By releasing the guilt that has haunted my past and embracing my present self—the self that struggles with fear and pain and uncertainty—I have a feeling this will also make a way toward strengthening my future. I want to fill my past, present, and future with love, compassion, grace, and forgiveness. But how?

Chapter 13

One Thing

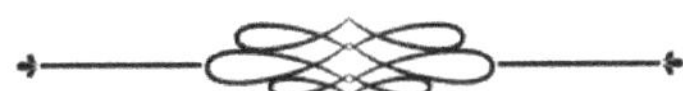

Fresh sea air fills my lungs as I step out of the camper van, and I allow myself to enjoy the butterflies of excitement inside. Anthony and I have been looking forward to this weekend getaway at Banna Beach for weeks, a chance to escape the daily grind and just be together. But as we set up our half-tent on the beach, I wonder how much my physical inability will affect our time here.

I try to push my worries aside as Anthony suggests a walk down the beach. I wrap a scarf tightly around my head and face, trying to shield myself from the biting wind. Still, it rushes toward me, causing my face to burn with pain. I knew this walk on the beach would be a challenge, with the unpredictable and harsh winds whipping against my sensitive skin. But I don't want to disappoint Anthony. I know he has been looking forward to this time together.

As we make our way down the beach, the sand crunching beneath my feet and the wind howling in my ears, I try to focus on my breathing to keep my mind off the pain flaring up in my face and legs. The wind is relentless, piercing my skin with a thousand needles and sending electric shocks through my body.

I tug on Anthony's arm, motioning for him to walk slower. He looks at me with concern. I know he is struggling to understand the extent of my pain. My husband has watched me suffer for over a year now, and he must be dealing with his own grief and loss over the woman I once was.

I set my focus to the steps ahead, taking in the vastness of the beach, the sand, and the dunes nearby, but all I can think about is the overwhelming pain consuming me.

I finally can't take it any longer.

"I know we've only been walking for a few minutes," I say, "but the wind is just too much for me." I can see the disappointment in Anthony's eyes, but I am dealing with my own pain and frustration, and I don't have the energy to put on a brave face for him.

As we make our way back, the wind seems to pick up, hitting us head on and causing me even more pain. Our tent is just a few hundred metres ahead, but I can't walk anymore. I clutch onto Anthony's jacket, tears streaming down my face.

"Please, let me rest here for a few minutes."

"Come on, Michele, we're almost there. Just a few more metres and you can rest in the beach tent." Anthony's voice is laced with frustration.

I can't move. I collapse onto the sand, curling into a ball to shield myself from the wind. I close my eyes and focus on the sound of the waves, the peaceful ebb and flow of the ocean, trying to find comfort in the midst of this pain.

Anthony sits by my side, his frustration and irritation palpable, but I can't bring myself to care.

"I don't understand why you can't walk anymore," Anthony says, his voice harsh. "We used to walk for miles on the beach together, now you can barely make it a few steps."

I look up at him, frustration mingling with guilt. "I'm sorry, Anthony. I know this isn't what you signed up for. But my stupid illness gets triggered with the wind and saps me of any energy I have. Can't you see?"

"You make it sound like I'm not supportive," Anthony retorts, his voice rising. "I'm here for you, but it's frustrating to see you like this. Can't you just push on?"

"What do you think I have been doing? I'm at my limit. My body feels like it's been put through a meat grinder." Tears wet my cheeks. "I feel guilty and frustrated for not being able to do the things we used to do together, but this is what it is, a stupid invisible illness that no one can see but that controls my life!"

We sit in silence for a few moments.

"You can keep walking if you like. I need some time before I can go any farther," I say.

Anthony stands up and lets out a sigh. "I just wish there was something I could do to help." He walks towards a driftwood log grounded on the sand. I focus on the waves, praying for the pain to subside so I can make my way back to the safety of my little tent.

About ten minutes later, the pain subsides enough for me to return to our beach tent. I curl into a foetal position, trying to escape the frustration of not being able to walk on the beach with my husband. I can tell he's irritated. Is it because I can't keep up or is he just tired of everything?

Anthony pokes his face into the tent after his walk. "You're only dealing with one thing; I'm the one trying to keep everything going!"

I sit up. "That one thing? Are you for real?!" I shout at him. His words have cut me deeper than the cold wind whipping around us.

"Yes, Michele, you only have to deal with your health. I'm the one dealing with everything else since you haven't been able to do anything." All his pent-up emotions are finally coming out right here in the middle of a windy day on the beach.

I burst into tears. This is almost worse than the physical pain. My husband has been with me through all of this, and his words make me feel so helpless. All the negative thoughts I've been suppressing come rushing to the forefront.

"You can't understand it. This 'one thing' is everything ... how can you say this?"

Anthony walks off and I'm left alone. So much for a nice break from it all.

When Anthony returns from his walk an hour later, I remain silent as we make our way to the caravan. He prepares a simple dinner, and I sit on the table across from him, looking outside at the other caravans and passersby. We are both silent in our own inner turmoil.

Finally, I break the silence. "Anthony, I need you to understand that this 'one thing'—my health—is my entire life! It's consumed every waking moment, every breath I take. The chronic pain, fatigue, and constant uncertainty of what my future holds, it's not just 'one thing.' You don't understand."

My voice breaks but I push through the tears. "You don't know what it's like to live with this pain every single day. What it's like to not know if I'll be able to even walk down the beach without a flare-up."

"You're right, I don't understand." Anthony's voice is heavy with sadness. "But I'm here for you. I *want* to understand and help you through this."

"It's not just about your help," I exclaim. "I need you to understand that my world is wrapped around this one thing. My health is gone, replaced with chronic pain and fatigue. I can't just snap out of it and move on with my life like nothing happened."

The tension in the air is thick as silence descends once more. I'm frustrated that he can't understand the extent of my pain and the constant battle I'm fighting every day.

The wind continues to howl outside our camper. *How can I expect anyone to truly understand the depth of my pain and the impact it has on my life?*

"If you can't seem to understand that this 'one thing' is everything for me, then I might as well be dead. It's only one thing, right? One DEATH. Done. Over with. How is that in comparison?" I sob, the emotions coming from a deep part of me where shame and guilt and fear linger in hiding.

"I just want you to be more interested in my life as well," Anthony says sheepishly.

"I *am* interested in your life. It's just a lot for me to take right now. I still don't know what my new self is supposed to do, how I'm supposed to navigate all of this."

I feel like I'm losing the person I love the most, but Anthony's words offer a window into his challenges. He must feel like he's being pushed to the sidelines because of this invisible illness that has taken front and centre stage in my life.

We're both fighting to find a way to support each other, but the weight of our individual struggles is all either of us can bear.

This 'one thing' has taken everything from both of us.

Chapter 14

Connecting with Little Me

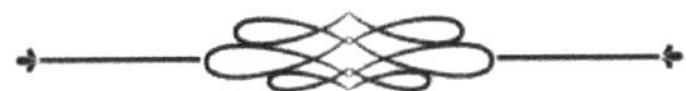

Tension clings to my body as I enter the dimly lit room. Hawaiian melodies waft through the air, weaving with the scent of a single, flickering candle. I'm nervous at the thought of the two-hour session that awaits me—a lomi lomi massage followed by a reiki session.

Will I find comfort through the sacred art? Or will it be yet another failed attempt at finding an avenue that provides healing? It's not just the physical pain that plagues me. Everything is weighing down on me all at once, and the journey toward healing itself feels almost as exhausting as the pain.

I've done everything right, gone down every medical avenue, experimented with countless medications. Now, I am grasping at straws for any semblance of relief in the realm of holistic methods. This Hawaiian massage technique is yet another recommendation on the long and winding path.

Marzena enters the room. "Are you comfortable, Michele?" She adjusts the sarong beneath me, her touch both gentle and unsettling.

"As much as I can be," I reply. Before surrendering to this session, I'd been grappling with the weight of my childhood abuse. The notion that the body keeps score haunts my thoughts. I've been seeing a new therapist, attempting to find relief by acknowledging that part of me that was abused. But truth be told, I want nothing more than to forget it ever happened. I'm not yet ready to face my inner traumas, terrified of my world crumbling beneath their weight—a world that already feels as if it's ready to implode.

My body is locked in pain—my face plagued by searing zaps, my legs hypersensitive to touch, and my lower back tense in what seems like an endless spasm. My fatigue is compounded by the weight of financial pressures. If I dare open up and peer inward, I fear I may drown.

"Let's take a few deep breaths," Marzena suggests, reaching beneath the table and pulling out a vial of lemongrass-scented oil. I try to focus on the scent and backdrop of music.

God, please help me find presence in this moment. I silently pray. *Please, grant me the serenity to relax.*

"That's better, Michele," Marzena observes. "I can sense your body gradually surrendering its grip on stress. Remember, this is your sanctuary. Remind yourself that these two hours are dedicated to relaxation, and I will do my utmost to aid you."

Her hands begin to coax the tension from my back and neck. "Is the pressure to your liking, or would you prefer something lighter?" Marzena's hands glide to my shoulders.

"That's fine," I mutter, closing my eyes. The music reminds me of waves crashing in the distance. *I am here for me*, I repeat silently, hoping to drown out the doubts that echo within. *This is my time to relax and allow myself to heal.*

The session progresses, Marzena's deft hands tracing delicate pathways across my legs and arms. I relax my arms and feel strain melting away from my neck and shoulders.

As the massage draws to a close, Marzena drapes a warm blanket over my body. I lie on my back, my eyes closed, a warm cloth resting upon them.

"Now, Michele, I want you to allow your body to reveal anything it might be holding onto. Don't fight it—simply let it be. Remember, this is your sanctuary."

Still uncertain, I try to open myself to the journey, whispering inwardly, *I am listening, body. Help me help you, please.*

Marzena's hands traverse different parts of my body. A surge of tension prickles within me as her hands graze my belly. I feel a wave of profound sadness, and I try to hold back the tears that threaten to spill forth.

"It's okay to release it, Michele. You're in a safe space," Marzena assures me.

In that instant, a memory grips me. I see myself as a child sitting on the cold floor, my back against the wall, crying, overwhelmed by shame and guilt for sharing the truth of my abuse.

The dam finally crumbles, and the tears flow freely.

"It's okay, Michele," Marzena's voice reaches me in this dark place. "Let it out."

I sob, feeling like a helpless child. Marzena continues to rest her hand gently on my belly. "You're doing so well, Michele. What can you see?"

"I can see my younger self—terrified, confused, and sad," I respond.

"Allow your younger self to see you. Let her know that you're there for her. Can you do that?" Marzena asks.

An otherworldly experience unfolds—I witness myself looking upon my younger self, our gazes locked, both brimming with tears, burdened by sorrow, shame, and guilt.

"Michele, can you hold your inner child's hand? Can you envision a safe place where both of you can find refuge?"

As tears stream down my face, I picture myself reaching out, clasping the hand of my inner child. Together, we walk toward the light, leaving behind the frigid room and the wall against which she once leaned. I envision us walking over white sand on a secluded beach, far removed from the hurts of the world.

It's just the two of us, wavy black hair whipped by an ocean breeze. I focus on our footprints marking the sand—one set the small steps of a child and the other, a woman farther along in the journey but finally returning to rescue her inner child from the place where she sat in secret for far too long.

"Now, tell her that you are here for Michele, that you are strong and resilient, and that you will protect her—the protection she longed for when she was younger," Marzena's voice reorients me to the present. I tune back into my body, feeling Marzena's hand firmly on my belly. Her other hand glides from my back to my head, as though she is holding my emotions and body in a delicate balance.

"Find comfort together, Michele. Can you do that?" Once again, I immerse myself in the vision. A blue sky stretches endlessly above us. I walk hand in hand with my younger self, allowing us both to shed the weight of anguish and replace it with connection and beauty.

The Hawaiian melodies continue in the background, Marzena's hands alternating between my head and shoulders, as if guiding me back to a state of self-assurance within my own skin. The session draws to a close.

"You did exceptionally well, Michele. Take your time rising and always remember that you have this safe haven to retreat to." Marzena lights incense and then exits the room. The sharp fragrance of lemongrass fills the air, and I know it will always serve as a reminder of the journey I embarked upon to free my inner child.

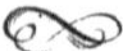

There are stories I have woven to conceal my trauma to make it more palatable to myself and, perhaps, to others who might hear my stories. Finally, I have reached the point where I am willing to embark on this journey of healing. It's about facing the feelings of rejection, confusion, and uncertainty that have plagued me, recognizing that beneath these layers lies a fundamental question of self-worth.

I am determined to delve into the depths of these struggles, mindful not to judge anyone along the way. I am fully aware that it will be a challenging process, but I begin to understand how these traumatic experiences have taken hold of my body, mind, and spirit—how they have shaped me. To reprogram myself, to update the very software of my being, I must expel the viruses, trojans, and other impediments that have cluttered and slowed down my metaphorical "computer system."

I need a reboot.

Returning home after the therapy session, I journal about the experience. I do not want to miss any part of what I have experienced. I begin to write:

My journey inward with the help of my therapist is opening different parts of me that I have shunned, like my younger self—little Michele—whom in some way or another I have kept at arm's length, holding her responsible for my mistakes and traumas.

I feel a metamorphosis deep within, a newfound lightness awakening my senses and unearthing a forgotten part of myself. Though seemingly small, my inner child carries monumental significance. I turned away from her, but now I am learning to embrace her.

Being gentle with oneself is perplexing. I struggle to offer myself the same love and understanding I extend to others. That little girl was blameless, naïve. She was simply a child, but this older version of myself has been condemning her. Did she know any better? No. It's time to offer her the love she deserves.

Now, in my late thirties, I am finally confronting my deepest wounds. Beneath the layers of confidence and capability I've constructed lies a vulnerable core. I am afraid to peel back the protective covering. Do I retract and retreat? Or do I immerse in these emotions, trusting that I will be guided through this journey? I continue to write:

I pledge to surrender to this process, to flow with it, to embrace the healing I've postponed. I will nurture my own resilience, regardless of how long it takes. I will no longer suppress my inner child. I refuse to sacrifice my truth on the altar of false strength.

I am strong, simply by virtue of my existence. I have not surrendered to the darkness that has beckoned. And I will not surrender now.

As I pen these words, I affirm my commitment and allow myself to embrace the full range of emotions, including the guilt that still clings to me because of what took place in my past—standing in the aftermath with a burden no child should bear.

This is how I create space for healing, I write, *by allowing myself to feel the pain, by pouring love over the wounds. This is what I need, what I commit to giving myself.*

When dark memories come knocking, I grant myself a sacred "time out" to sit with my younger self, holding her tightly and offering my presence. I permit her tears to flow freely. I encourage her to voice her confusion, fear, and helplessness. I give her permission to reveal that she didn't know what to do, that her loyalty kept her silent, preventing her from seeking the help she needed.

Yes, this is what she needs. And this is what I need. A safe haven. In choosing to accept and open to my inner child, I also extend love to myself as I am today. I offer myself permission to find comfort in the little things—a therapeutic massage, a cup of hot chocolate, a long, soothing bath—allowing my senses to decompress and just be. To be at peace, at ease, and in harmony with the different parts of who I am.

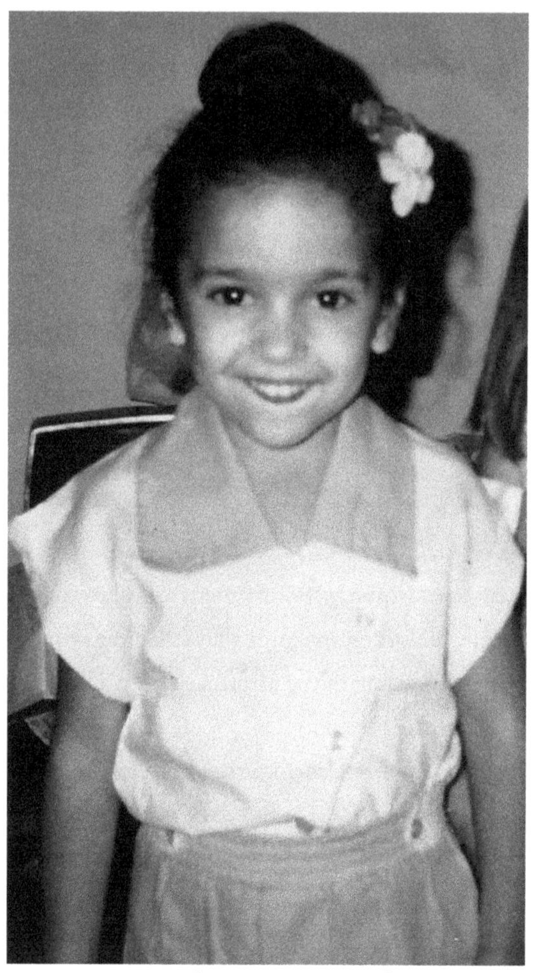

Londrina - PR - Brazil

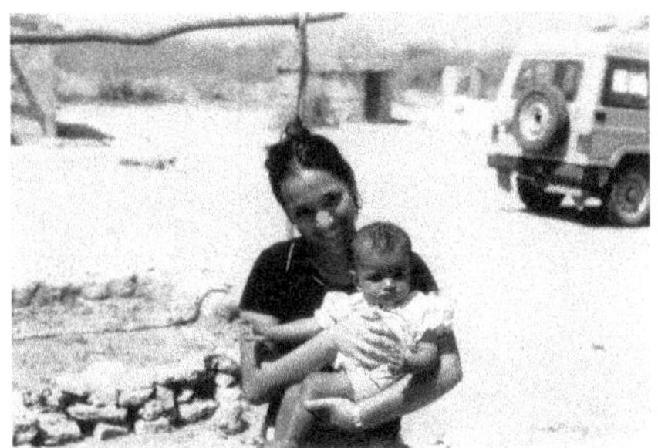

Gujarat - India

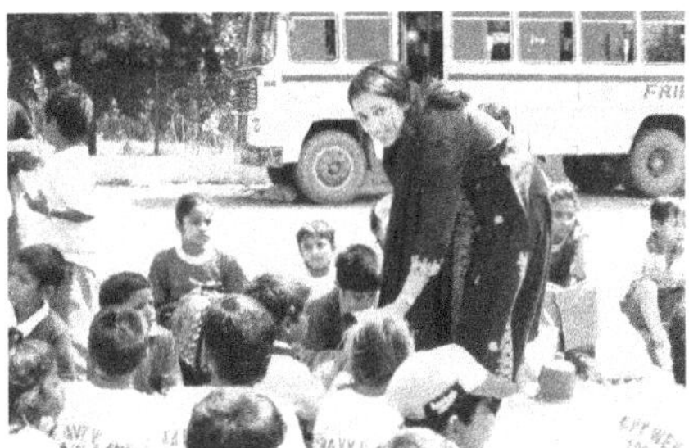

New Delhi - India

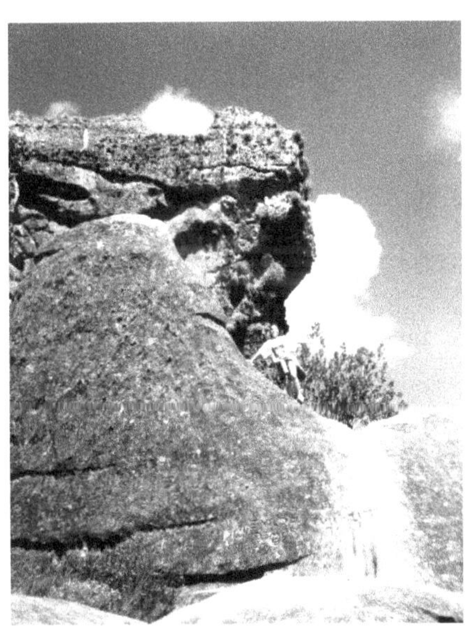

Parque Estadual de Vila Velha - Ponta Grossa - PR - Brazil

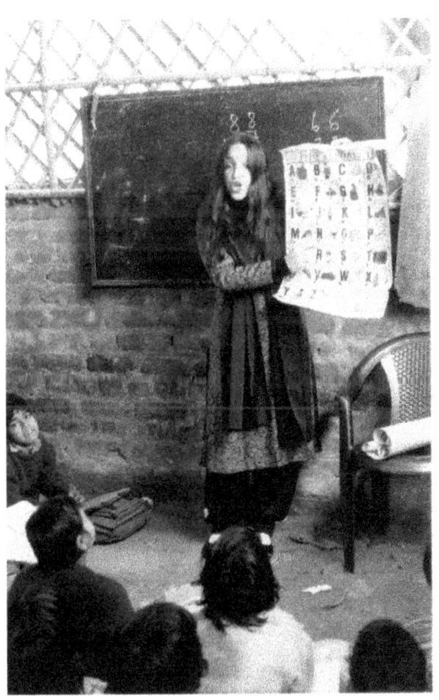

Gurgaon - Haryana - India

Part 3: Slow Acceptance

"When we truly embrace acceptance, that's when our body exhales and can begin healing."
– **Kris Carr**

Chapter 15

Acknowledging

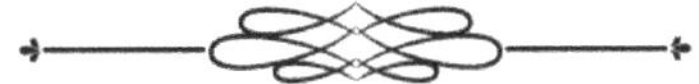

My friend has been asking me for weeks to go to a meditation session with her. While I enjoy guided meditation on my phone, attending an in-person session intimidates me. However, I've finally agreed.

As I follow her black BMW in my old blue Fiat Punto, I'm convinced I'll do something embarrassing. Maybe full-on ugly crying in front of a bunch of strangers. The drive itself is bad enough as we take winding one-way roads, pass by towering cathedrals and castles, and cross narrow bridges with oncoming traffic in Limerick City. By the time we drive out of the city, my heart is pounding and I'm ready to turn around and head back home.

As we drive further from the city, doubt starts to creep in. I don't know where we are going, and I don't like it. My friend turns into a pub parking area, and I follow her, surprised to find this is where we are meant to be. I would have preferred knowing the full route ahead of time.

As we ascend the stairs and enter a small yoga studio, we're greeted with warmth by a lady with straight black hair, a small build, and a big smile. She asks us to remove our shoes. We enter the yoga room, where about 30 chairs are set in place. A small statue of Buddha and a poster of the Tara Kadampa Meditation Centre adorn the front of the room. A table with refreshments and cups is on the right. Near the back of the room, I spot a table with books and CDs.

My friend and I sit next to each other, and I ground myself with a prayer. *God, please help me to listen with the ears of curiosity. Help me to learn something that can help me along my journey, please.* I watch the different people coming into the room and am comforted by the diversity of the group.

The main speaker talks about different forms of acceptance and surrendering, then guides us through a meditation practice. I'm still struggling to accept the thought that I'm going to be sick for who knows how long. But the speaker's guided meditation strikes a chord with me.

"Make peace with whatever you are struggling with," he says. The room is silent. Probably each person sitting around me is also reflecting on those words and how the advice fits their personal situation. Because my struggle is with pain, I keep asking myself, *Peace with pain? But how?*

The meditation practice isn't easy. It triggers a few very strong pain surges throughout my body, and I have to take some very deep breaths. I feel like I'm breathing in all the dust particles that have been settling in this room since who knows when and start coughing. It develops into a full-on coughing fit. *I knew I was going to do something embarrassing.*

I try to hold my breath and control my coughing. When this doesn't work, I head to the bathroom with a glass of water, hoping that people won't hear me in there. But the whole room is silent, and the bathroom is just two doors down the hall. I'm sure they hear me hacking away. Tears stream down my face as I try to regulate myself, telling my body that I'm not asphyxiating and that there's enough air to breathe. I eventually get my coughing under control and refill my glass of water in the bathroom.

When I return to the room, all eyes are on me. I quickly take my seat, trying to get back into the rhythm of the class. When the class ends, I speak to the gentleman leading the course and explain to him about my diagnosis and how hard it is for me to accept it.

"I feel that if I accept it, I will be surrendering to it, which might make me fall into depression because I won't be fighting it anymore." I am surprised at how quickly I feel ready to be honest with him. Maybe those sessions with my therapist are doing some good after all.

He looks intently at me and asks, "What if you were to accept that you have this diagnosis and not resist it but see it as a gift? What are the good things that you might see from it?"

He's good at this. His question gets straight to the heart of the matter. What "gift" might I find in this whole ordeal? I process aloud. "Well, I've been home more, and I get to see my kids. Before, I was constantly on the road for my job and didn't have much time with them." I'm still unsure as to how that's going to help me.

"Well, that is a very good thing," he agrees. "Accepting doesn't mean you're giving up the hope to find healing. Accepting and surrendering means you're not resisting but letting things play out while looking at the good things coming to you. In your case, you can spend more time with your family, and while it's probably very difficult to have a debilitation, there is a lot of good that can come from this place."

I thank him. Now that I've been here, maybe it's not so bad. Maybe I'll come to the next class. His teachings feel like they hold some key in learning how to accept my situation.

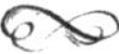

Back at home, the clock ticks loudly in the background; each second passing feels like a lost opportunity. *Why is this so hard?* I sit here, not knowing how to just let it all go. Life is happening without my permission. I'm exhausted by the constant struggle in my mind between my ideas of how things should be and how things are actually playing out.

I feel powerless, and I don't like it.

I always strive to be the best at everything I do. I give 110% of myself to every task, planning everything to perfection. But now, my reality is far removed from my expectations.

While rummaging through some old papers, I come across something I'd written a few years back, projecting what my life should be like by my 40th birthday. On the list: speaking French and Italian fluently, playing the piano and guitar very well, having an amazing bikini body, and travelling around the world as a public speaker. All this seems so far-fetched now. I'm 38 years old and the things I thought I would have achieved by now seem to be a distant dream.

I recently attempted to review my French with my son using the Michael Thomas method, but my brain couldn't handle it. I may have time, but these days it feels like my mental capacity is sorely limited, and I become overwhelmed easily.

Forget traveling the world as a public speaker; simple tasks such as making the bed, inviting a friend over for coffee, or keeping my house tidy leave me exhausted. My pain increases when I overexert myself, and nagging thoughts begin once more—haunting me, telling me I'm not good enough.

How do I let go? How do I accept that I can't do everything I want to do? Like I told the meditation director, part of me feels that accepting my limitations is succumbing to my condition, accepting that I'll never get better. And I don't want to never get better.

But maybe accepting it will help me feel less like a tight coil wound up in knots. What if I could accept that doing five percent of something is still *something*?

Releasing my grip on things is like untying those knots, but each one requires time and patience and focus. A book that my friend Mindy lent me is a real eye opener, describing the Japanese Kaizen method. I turn to the Kaizen method, which encourages taking small, gradual steps forward to help me navigate my reality.

This approach of constant improvement makes me think of tending to a garden, carefully nurturing each plant to reach its full potential. It's okay to have a variety of spaces in my life that are like little saplings, plants that are not yet deeply rooted, vines that aren't yet growing fruit. It's okay to struggle and not have everything figured out, to embrace the journey and hopefully, gradually, along the way find peace with what I cannot change.

I have been stuck in a desert for far too long, denying that anything is wrong, refusing to give in to my body's needs.

Now, finally, I am beginning to acknowledge the truth.

I am ill. I am in pain. And I cannot control it.

This invisible illness is trying to teach me lessons, but they are bitter pills to swallow—learning to go slow, to accept that my reality is different now. Things I used to do in my spare time—making my bed, cleaning my home, doing laundry—now require *all* my focus and energy.

But I am learning to appreciate completing these tasks as small victories, to take joy in the act of doing rather than in the end result.

If time is the most precious gift we have—and people wiser than me say that it is—then I have squandered too much of it fretting about things beyond my control. Now, I just want to be present in each moment, to savour the time I have with my family, to read a good book and enjoy it rather than rushing through it. These small pleasures have become my refuge, my respite from the pain and fatigue that plague me.

It's not easy, though. Every day is a battle to accept that I cannot control everything. I cannot control my illness, but I can control how I react to it. I can choose to see the beauty in the present moment. I am slowly learning to let go of my need for control and embrace the uncertainty of life.

Chapter 16

Daffodils and New Chapters

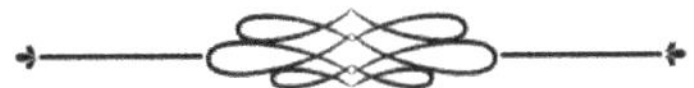

Raindrops trickle from roofs, the sound bringing comfort. We are on vacation in Algarve, Portugal, and I find myself drawn to the natural beauty of this place. A light breeze carries the faint aroma of pine from nearby trees. I am reminded of the good things in life, such as the sun, sand, and sea. It's a welcome change to my usual surroundings.

Three more days here, and then we return to Ireland. It would be great to get more sun, and I hope the rain stops soon.

Earlier today, Anthony and I took a walk on the cliffs surrounding Praia da Maria Luisa. Overlooking the beach are some cute houses. We daydreamed together about how wonderful it would be to have *that* view, *that* pool, walks on *that* beach. We talked about owning one of those small Portuguese-looking white walls with terracotta roof tiles overlooking the ocean, with clay pots around the backyard and low branches of old trees creating shade.

My pain has been considerably less here than in Ireland. A home away from home in Portugal would be heaven on earth and a dream come true. The sun, beach, and change of scenery have been refreshing and helped refuel my energy levels. The thought of leaving and going back home, where I am usually in severe pain, is hard to ignore.

It's the sixth of November 2020. Two years ago today, I had my first experience of nerve pain that brought me to my knees, literally. I've been off work for two years, learning to live with an invisible illness. It has been a slow two years, yet at the same time, it feels like it has gone by too fast. An eternity. A moment.

To be honest, I'm frustrated that I have nothing tangible to show for these past two years. I haven't been working or receiving a promotion, as would have been the case if everything had remained normal. Most of the time, I've been stuck at home.

When people see me and ask, "Are you still sick? Because you look great!" it's a compliment that stabs me in the heart. What they can't see is the pain that keeps me awake at night and envelops me in a thick cloud. I have to force myself to walk, to create movement so the rest of my body doesn't suffer and remain inert because of my neuralgia. Tears stream down my face whenever I do my exercise, yoga, or Pilates.

Any type of movement takes effort, and no one can see that! Not even my doctor. He sees me physically, and I look normal and healthier than most patients my age. These other patients aren't doing what I'm doing—intermittent fasting, juicing, drinking lots of water, and watching their diet. I try so hard to give my body what it needs in the hope it will get my brain wires sending the proper signals soon.

It's a constant fight to keep in shape. Even these two weeks of holidays have been difficult in their own way. Invisible illness is hard; how do I explain something to others that is impossible to make sense of myself? The fatigue, tiredness, and lack of energy have affected my desire to do things I once would have jumped to do. This year has been challenging for everyone due to the pandemic, but for me, it's been especially tough.

Yet as I take stock of all that happened in these last two years, I can begin to see I have been learning to live with my limitations, adjusting to my new reality. Not easy, but necessary. Acceptance is the first step towards healing—and I am slowly moving in that direction.

The tension increases every winter. The cold, humid air of Ireland cuts through my bones, making the pain levels almost unbearable. I dream of moving to a warmer climate, at least during the winter months. The idea of finding relief in a place where the sun shines and the air is dry is incredibly tempting.

I imagine myself in Portugal, soaking up the sun, my body warmed and my spirits lifted by the extra dose of endorphins. Just being in such a lovely place with higher levels of vitamin D could make a world of difference.

But reality pulls me back. My family, my boys' schooling, our friends, and my doctors are all in Ireland. The idea of uprooting our lives and starting over in another country is unrealistic. Would the boys adapt to a new school? Would I find doctors who understand my condition?

Besides the logistics and emotional toll of such a change, I can't take too much heat. Anything over 28 degrees Celsius, and I'm hit with debilitating migraines. Finding that perfect, even temperature feels like an elusive dream. The balance I need is so delicate—warm enough to ease my pain but cool enough to avoid triggering migraines.

For now, I'll cherish these last few days and the small relief this environment brings, knowing that each moment of warmth is a gift.

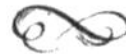

I sit at my desk, typing on my computer. It's a rare morning of peace and quiet, something that's been in short supply lately after the busyness of the 2020 holiday season. I take a break from the keyboard and my mind automatically drifts to the constant ache that's been throbbing through my body and increasing since the pandemic hit.

Being stuck at home due to the lockdown has made managing my chronic pain even more difficult. The things that used to bring me comfort and relief have been taken away—the soothing touch of my massage therapist, the precise needles of my acupuncturist, the encouragement and exercises from my physiotherapist, and the heat and warmth I would get from the sauna and jacuzzi at my local gym.

An upcoming visit with my neurologist has been indefinitely postponed, leaving me anxious about when I'll be able to get the care I need to manage my condition. The burning sensation in my cheek and running down my jaw is a constant reminder of my struggle. Thankfully, at least the sessions with my psychologist can be held online.

It's not just the physical pain that's weighing me down. The emotional impact of the pandemic is taking its toll on me, too. I know this is what many are dealing with right now, but I miss spending time with my friends, and I feel trapped in my own home. The only person I'm allowed to see is my sister, who's in my support bubble. She's a single parent of three, and her younger boys are roughly the same age as my sons.

I hear my boys bickering in the other room. They're also struggling with the restrictions and uncertainty brought on by the pandemic, and it's hard to know how to support them when I'm struggling to cope. I take a deep breath and try to shake off the heaviness that's been weighing me down. I'm doing my best to stay strong and take care of my family, but it's hard when I feel like I should be the one receiving care.

Shifting in the chair to ease my sciatic pain, I rub my temples in hopes of melting away some tension. The sun feels warm on my skin, and I'm grateful for this small moment of peace. I know I need to keep pushing through, even when it feels like everything is stacked against me.

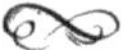

My husband enters the room and throws open the curtains. "There is a fresh layer of snow from last night, the first snowfall of the year!" I push back the covers and step to the bay window. The sun is barely visible even though it is 9:30 in the morning, and dark grey clouds drift across the sky.

A thin layer of snow has fallen, covering surfaces in a dusting of white. The road outside is beautiful. A neighbour is playing with her little boys in the snow. Although there isn't enough to build a snowman, it's still a lovely sight.

Despite the cold weather that usually triggers my pain, I venture outdoors, bundled up in my thick-down, brown jacket with a sheepskin hood. I also pull on a black balaclava, which only allows my eyes to be seen. I open the front door and let the sun carry me outside, taking in the beauty of the snow-covered landscape.

The snow crunching beneath my feet brings a smile to my face. *I just need to be in the moment.* I walk back to the house and notice my phone in its red case, which my husband had brought downstairs. I grab it and walk back outside, wanting to document this moment.

My husband is ready to go for a walk with Lady, our dog. Changing the aperture settings on my phone, I capture Lady's pawprints on the snow. I face the sun, feeling the warm rays on the little bit of my face that is exposed, and set out with my husband.

As we slowly make our way down the block, my husband asks, "You sun tanning?"

"I am trying to stay in the moment here." I smile. "I suppose I am sun tanning, through my many layers."

We turn right, toward the main road. The driveways of our neighbours are completely covered in a white sheet of snow. I capture more snaps, including a bird print in the snow and a shot of my husband and Lady waiting patiently a few paces ahead.

The houses on the left block the sun, and my legs start to feel very cold. Despite being wrapped up, I feel a twinge of pain beneath my eyes, which I know will trigger more pain. *What should I do?* My husband looks back at me standing between the side road and the main road.

"Are you done with your walk?" he asks.

"Yes, I think I need to turn back." The snow crunches beneath my feet as I retrace my steps. I hear the faint sound of birds chirping in the distance and try to spot them but they're too smart to be out in the cold. The sound of cars going up and down the main road is distant enough to not intrude on this little space of peace.

This is being present; this is enjoying the moment.

I stand in my driveway and marvel at a daffodil that has already begun to sprout. Its vibrant golden petals peek through the snow, pushing against winter's icy grip. I see it as a symbol of hope, a reminder that despite the cold and the darkness, spring is on its way.

But as I look around, I see nothing but snow and sleet, as if the daffodil has gotten the seasons all mixed up. "Looks like you got the wrong memo," I mutter, feeling a little silly talking to a flower.

As I retreat to the warmth of my home, the ache in my bones grows stronger. I slump down onto the couch, too tired to even take off my jacket and balaclava. Pain threatens to overwhelm me, but I try to keep in mind the things I've been learning about acceptance and surrender. I focus on the good things I've experienced so far today, hoping to push the pain to the back of my mind.

Distraction is my go-to strategy, and I quickly send the picture of the daffodil to my mom, uncle, and a friend.

My friend responds right away. “It’s a lovely symbol,” she writes. “The first sign of spring and new hope.”

I take a deep breath and repeat a mantra to myself. “May I enjoy each moment. May I be present. May I be here.”

In this moment, surrounded by warmth and love, I know that everything will be okay. The pain may linger, but so too will hope and resilience.

May I be like the daffodil.

Chapter 17

A Delicate Dance

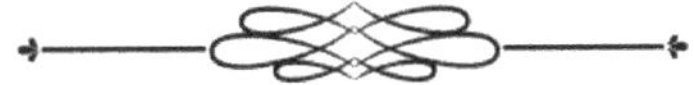

I receive a medical exemption from wearing a mask because of the pain it triggers on my already sensitive face. But not wearing a mask in public during the pandemic brings its own set of problems. I navigate a delicate dance between self-preservation and societal expectations.

I visit Crescent Shopping Mall in Limerick, deliberately unmasked. Sunlight filters through glass ceilings, brightening the bustling scene below. The air is tinged with a mixture of scents—perfume wafting from a nearby cosmetic store, freshly brewed coffee from a café tucked in a corner, and the mouth-watering aroma of pastries emanating from a bakery. The atmosphere is charged with the pulse of hurried footsteps, the murmur of conversations, and occasional laughter echoing through the atrium.

Shops adorned with vibrant displays beckon. Navigating this sensory overload, I encounter a stern-faced security guard who intercepts my path. "Where is your mask?" he demands.

I stand as tall as my stature allows. "I am exempt," I state firmly, raising my right hand. The security guard's initial sternness softens, and he offers a prompt apology. The triumph is subtle, a ripple in the sea of masked faces around me.

Later, the cinema becomes the stage for a different act. A lanky man dressed in black stands at the entrance. The lighting is dim, and I breathe in the scent of buttered popcorn. The theatre is a reprieve from countless weeks of being homebound.

The man's gaze fixes on my husband, a tall figure exuding strength. As his eyes shift to me—a small figure with brown skin, conspicuously maskless—I feel the tension heighten.

"Put on your mask," he commands.

"I am exempt," I manage to say. His eyes narrow in disbelief, and a familiar sense of insignificance envelops me. "I have a medical exemption," I say firmly. "But it's private medical information; I won't be showing it to you." I stride past him with my boys following behind me.

Anthony, sensing my unease, squeezes my hand. "Don't waste energy on him. He's just on a power trip." His words soothe me, but the encounter with the lanky man leaves me drained. Knees trembling, I settle into my seat. The movie begins, distracting me from the internal echoes of the confrontation. I finally immerse myself in the movie with my family.

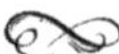

In an online session with my therapist, I share my experiences with the mall security guard and the cinema attendant. Both encounters ignited a desire within me to assert myself. As we dive into a discussion about boundaries, she suggests a visual exercise, guiding me to extend my hands in front of me.

"Now leave one hand thrust outward. Make a clear 'stop' signal. This indicates the need to avoid overextension," she explains. I follow her instructions. "Turn the other hand inward, inviting introspection."

This gesture she teaches me reflects the delicate balance I aim for between asserting myself and avoiding unnecessary conflict.

Recalling my confrontation at the mall, I recall instinctively putting my hand up, palm facing outward—a shield against the intrusion on my mask-exempt status. Outstretched hands symbolise vigilance, reminding me to recognize and respect my boundaries.

In this virtual session, guided by my therapist, I rotate clockwise with my hands still extended, forming a protective circle around myself—a tangible assertion of my personal sanctuary.

"This is Michele's space. Back off," she declares. "It's okay, you can say that."

I say it aloud, cracking a smile. "This is Michele's space. Back off." I move my arms to the right and left, forming a semi-circle around me. My left hand faces my surroundings—a tapestry of objects and souvenirs around my home office. My right hand faces inward, and my therapist prompts me to notice the intricate lines etched upon my palm.

After the session, I sit in solitude. I look at my hands—symbols of my boundaries and self-protection. I have the power to transform them into a source of strength—a tribute to my authentic voice and the belief that I deserve to be heard.

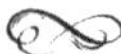

Putting into practice my stance on assertiveness and listening to my body comes with its challenges. Finally, I am able to travel. At the airport in Faro, Portugal, I stand out as the lone figure without a mask, waltzing through the airport. Two authoritative police officers approach me with stern gazes.

"Sua mascara." The officer points to my face, halting me in my tracks.

"I am exempt," I reply in English, hoping to move past them. However, their towering figures and decisive stance make it clear that I cannot proceed until they are satisfied.

"Excuse me, Ma'am, can I see your mask exemption documentation?"

My mind races as panic sets in. Fumbling through my phone, I search for the letter. A feeling of vulnerability envelops me, accompanied by a sense of hopelessness. Perhaps it's the authority these figures display?

One of the officers exudes an overwhelming sense of power. In that moment, I feel my body shrink, my back slouch, and my knees weaken. I become a mere shadow of myself, belittled and vulnerable. I feel as if these men might whisk me away to an isolated room, where I would be trapped indefinitely.

My mind becomes a whirlwind of thoughts and fears in those few harrowing minutes. I try to locate the letter on my phone while a dizzying sensation grips me, threatening to unleash a full-blown panic attack.

The officer becomes impatient. "We need to verify your exemption. Please find the documentation quickly." His hands rest on his hips in a superman pose.

The overwhelming presence of authority triggers something dark within, transporting me back to times when I felt defenceless and vulnerable. *Keep calm. Find the letter. You're an adult now; you can handle this,* I tell myself, scrolling through my phone in search of the letter. After what feels like an eternity, I present the letter with trembling hands.

The first police officer inspects the letter. Then his partner takes my phone and reads it. They exchange glances and the more imposing of the two finally says, "Alright, you can proceed." Relief washes over me, but the emotional residue lingers.

As I navigate through the airport, the line for security and metal detection looms ahead. Another security guard approaches, demanding, "Mask, please."

"Here we go again," I mutter to myself, attempting to breathe. At least I already have the letter pulled up on my phone. I show it to him.

The process repeats—*seven times.* Each encounter heightens my anxiety, triggering memories of childhood vulnerability. The boarding pass scan, the security line, and finally the passport control—all fraught with the struggle to maintain composure.

I can't believe how much energy each of these exchanges takes from me! I don't know what is worse, having to explain myself and prove my mask exemption, or the deeper trigger—setting me on the verge of a panic attack. I am an adult, but my emotions are that of a scared child trying not to be scolded by yet another person.

I am walking in my truth, managing my pain the best I can, but all I feel is the sense of being judged, of being less than, of being wrong. It depletes me to the core.

The journey through the airport chips away my resilience with every judgmental gaze and every unspoken question. *Is it worth it?*

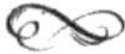

Before the online therapy session begins, I already feel depleted. I wear polka-dot pyjamas and hug a hot water bottle to ease the frustration.

As I recount the airport incident, Anne's empathy becomes a lifeline, stitching together the narrative of my past and present. "Michele, can you trace back to the first time you felt this vulnerable next to authority figures?"

The floodgates open, and I find myself transported to a time when I was a frightened little girl, defenceless against those in power. The trauma has etched itself into the core of my being, making authority figures loom like shadows capable of inflicting harm. With each probing question, Anne helps me draw connections between my present vulnerability and the scars of childhood abuse.

"Michele, it sounds like the airport triggered that deep-seated vulnerability from your childhood. The fear of not being able to protect yourself is still very much alive in those moments."

"Yes," I acknowledge. "It feels like I'm that frightened little girl again."

"I am sorry you feel this way, but I want you to know, you have done nothing wrong. You are fully within your right to exercise your mask exemption and take care of your health. I want you to hear me saying this, Michele." Her words are comforting, and I hug my hot water bottle even tighter.

"I know I have that right, but I just feel judged, as if I am the one on the wrong side of things." I open yet another layer of raw emotions. "It makes me feel like a scared, weak child."

"Michele, can you visualise that younger version of yourself?" Anne asks. "What does she need to hear from you right now?"

Closing my eyes, I picture myself as a little girl, frightened and fragile. Her dark curly hair and tear-stained face look up at me. I hold her hand and bring her into an embrace. "I'm here, sweetheart. I won't let anyone hurt you. You are strong, and I will protect you. We have the power now. We are not alone."

As I speak those words, Anne encourages me to place my hands over my heart, grounding myself in the present.

"Feel the warmth of your hands, Michele. This is your strength, your resilience. You've carried this little girl through so much and you continue to do so. It's incredible how strong you are. You built these layers of protection to survive. But now, we're peeling them back, layer by layer, so you can connect with the essence of who you are without the weight of the past."

Sharing this experience with Anne brings immense comfort. Her gentle questions open doors to understanding the coping mechanisms I developed to navigate a world that often feels hostile. There is much more to unravel, but I can discern the origin of these emotions.

I acknowledge my responsibility to help my younger self navigate through these triggers, not alone, but with me. By showing up for myself and embracing that adult side of me, I am essentially assisting her in regaining her confidence and self-assurance.

These are the fragments of myself that are slowly healing by being brought into the light. While grappling with this illness, I have been given an opportunity to explore the aspects of my body and mind that have lain "dis-eased" for far too long. This is part of my journey, and I trust that I will discover the healing my body, mind, and soul so desperately seek.

Progress is one step at a time, one moment at a time. It involves consistently moving in the right direction, placing one foot in front of the other, all the while trusting that I am here for all parts of myself. Being assertive is just one more step towards healing.

Chapter 18

Learning to Live with Pain

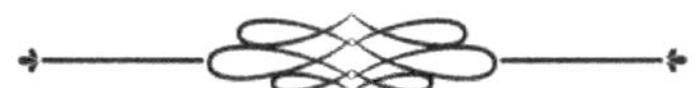

I sit quietly, reflecting on what my therapist said in the session that just ended. Her words echo what different people keep telling me, that I need to befriend my pain. I'm trying to come to terms with the idea but still struggle with it. Today, thinking about the concept has brought me to tears.

Pain is a strange and unwelcome guest that I don't want to invite into my life. It's a thorn in my side, a constant reminder of my limitations. Why on earth would I befriend it? But as I sit on my brown couch by the bay window, I realise that maybe pain is trying to tell me something. Maybe it's trying to help me, not harm me. The more I resist it, the more it persists. There must be a reason for this.

"I don't want to embrace pain," I say to myself. "I want it far, far, away from me."

But my therapist's words echo in my mind. *Allow yourself to acknowledge the pain. Listen to it. Befriend it.*

I take a deep breath and try to imagine pain as a person, sitting across from me. What would pain tell me if it could talk?

I'm here to help you, Pain whispers. *I'm not your enemy. I'm your ally.*

I don't want to believe it, but I know deep down it's true. I've been fighting against pain for months, refusing to acknowledge it, refusing to give it space in my life. But in doing so, I've only made things worse.

The judgmental part of my mind takes over. *You're not accomplishing anything with this pain in your life. You're a bad wife, a bad mother, a bad person.*

I can't escape the constant barrage of negative thoughts.

Maybe it is time to listen to pain instead of the harsh judgment of my own mind. Time to give myself permission to rest. To sleep in, to take a break, to not worry about the laundry or the dishes or the to-do list. It's hard silencing the inner critic, but I know it's what I need.

I recline on my couch, reminding myself that it's okay to move at a snail's pace. It's okay to take small steps instead of trying to do everything at once. It's okay to give myself a bit of love instead of beating myself up for not being perfect.

"I'm not perfect," I say out loud. "And that's okay."

I take a deep breath and let the words sink in. It's a hard truth to accept, but one that's essential for my healing. I may not be able to control the pain, but I can control how I respond to it. And right now, I choose to befriend it, to listen to it, and to embrace this journey, one step at a time.

I close my eyes. My mind travels back to an experience several years ago, before my illness, a rare day out with my husband and boys—just living and loving life.

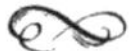

The sun is shining brightly on a gorgeous summer day as we embark on our first hike up the Sugar Loaf in Bray, Co. Wicklow. The boys dart ahead, their laughter echoing through the trees as they climb and explore. I smile, adjusting my hat and glasses, feeling the familiar excitement of going on another adventure with my family.

My comfortable hiking boots crunch against the gravel path as we begin our ascent.

"Wait up, boys!" I call, though I know they won't slow down. Their energy is boundless, and it brings me joy to see them so full of life.

My husband walks beside me, his backpack stuffed with a picnic lunch and our hiking essentials. He grins at me, a knowing look that says he's just as eager for this adventure as I am. We've always loved these hikes, these moments where the world feels open and endless.

"Think we'll make it to the top before lunch?" he asks, glancing up at the peak that seems to touch the sky.

"Absolutely," I reply. "We've got this."

Though we usually tackle Keeper Hill as our Christmas tradition, and explore different hikes around Ireland throughout the year, this is our first time on Sugar Loaf. The trail is a mix of rocky paths and verdant patches, and the air is filled with the scents of pine and earth.

As we climb, I notice the way the light filters through the trees, casting dappled shadows on the ground. The higher we go, the more breathtaking the view.

"Look, Mum! I'm king of the mountain!" my youngest son shouts from a nearby boulder, striking a triumphant pose.

I laugh. "Careful up there! Don't go too far ahead."

The climb gets steeper, and I can feel the burn in my muscles. The boys slow down just enough for us to catch up, their faces flushed. We keep a steady pace, enjoying the journey as much as the destination.

Finally, after an hour and a half, we reach the top. The sea stretches out in a vast expanse of blue on one side, while rolling hills and lush greenery spread out on the other. The breeze is cool and refreshing, a perfect reward for our effort.

"Isn't it amazing?" I take a deep breath, savouring the crisp air.

My husband nods. "Have you ever seen such a clear blue sky?"

We squeeze together on the summit for a few pictures, then Anthony pulls out our lunch and we sit together, sharing sandwiches and stories. The boys are still buzzing with energy, pointing out distant landmarks and marvelling at the height.

I lean back, feeling a deep sense of contentment.

As we prepare to descend, I take one last look at the view, committing it to memory. This is who I am, who we are—a family that embraces the beauty of nature and the thrill of adventure.

"That is who I want to be again," I whisper into the quiet afternoon. But how? Perhaps it is time to surrender to a deeper journey of self-discovery...

What parts of "me" make me who I am? Why do I do the things I do?

These questions have always plagued me, but I usually swept them into the darkest corners of my mind. In the past, I was able to avoid these reflective, contemplative matters by keeping busy. Now I have no recourse but to look honestly and openly at ... *me*.

Days like that gorgeous hike with my family to the summit of a mountain were few and far between. But why? I cast around for answers.

I remember the pride I felt when I graduated from university—the accolades and the thrill of climbing the career ladder. I threw myself into my work, completely consumed by it and often neglecting my husband and children.

I couldn't let anything, or anyone, hold me back. So determined was I to escape from dark memories and make up for past mistakes that I became heavily involved in my charitable organisation involving weekly visitations to elderly homes. I was a driving force behind the success of our "Adopt a Grandfriend" programme.

I was so proud of these accomplishments, but my drive to succeed overshadowed the most important people in my life—my husband and my boys. The irony is not lost on me that, in trying to escape my past, I only succeeded in trapping myself in a cycle of self-inflicted suffering.

As the memories of my past and the ghosts of my accomplishments wend their way through my consciousness, I make a commitment: I am determined to spend my time wisely, making things right and finding peace within myself for my sake and the sake of my family.

Chapter 19

Changing Times

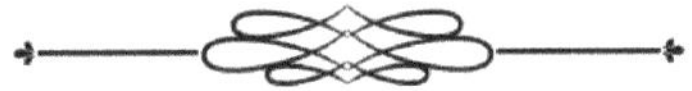

The car ride to Villiers Secondary School in Limerick is quiet, save for the hum of the engine and the occasional sniffle from Ryan in the backseat. My heart aches as I glance at him in the rearview mirror, his eyes wide and anxious.

"Mom, do you think I'll make friends quickly?"

"Of course you will, Honey," I say, trying to inject confidence into my voice. "You're a wonderful boy, and everyone will see that."

Next to him, my eldest rolls his eyes playfully. "Don't worry, Ryan. You'll be fine. Just avoid the cafeteria meatloaf."

It is August of 2021 and the school looms ahead, its gates wide open, welcoming students back after what feels like an eternity with the pandemic. The building stands tall, its brick walls still sturdy after 200 years of history. As we pull into the parking lot and step out of the car, the chatter of other families fills the air. I sense the mixed emotions of parents giving last-minute advice and kids laughing nervously.

I stretch, feeling the familiar twinge of pain in my back. I try to hide it, not wanting the boys to worry about me. They have enough to worry about. Ryan clings to his backpack, his knuckles white. Collin nudges him. "Come on, Ryan. Let's go check out the dorms and choose our beds first."

I smile, watching them interact. "Don't forget your bags," I remind them, my voice steady despite the knot in my stomach. We unload the car, and I help Ryan with his blankets.

As they gather their bags—bulky with bedding, pillows, sheets, and schoolbooks—I feel a pang of sadness. Due to the lingering COVID restrictions, I can't go inside with them. I can't see their rooms, can't help them set up. I stand by the car, watching as Collin confidently leads Ryan toward the boarding rooms. He turns back and grins.

"Mom, Ryan will be fine. I'll make sure of it."

I nod, swallowing the lump in my throat. "Thanks, Collin. Ryan, call me if you need anything, okay?"

Ryan glances back, his eyes a mix of nerves and excitement. "I will, Mom. Love you."

"Love you too, sweetheart," I say, my voice barely holding steady. "Both of you."

I watch them disappear into the building, my heart heavy. I take a deep breath, the cool morning air filling my lungs. The scent of freshly cut grass mingles with the distant aroma of the school's cafeteria breakfast wafting through the open doors.

Back in the car, the emptiness hits me hard. My mind races with worries about Ryan. Will he make friends? Will the kids be nice to him, or will he have problems with bullying? The thought of him facing challenges without me there to help makes my heart ache even more. And then there's Collin, stepping into his third year. He's more experienced, but I still worry. The drive home is quiet, the silence amplifying my fears and the dull ache in my body.

Once home, I stand in the living room, feeling the oppressive silence. I try to distract myself with my dog, Lady, but everything feels heavy and pointless. Just making my bed is a struggle, the pain in my body making every movement an effort.

When my boys are home, their presence pushes me to get up, to be strong for them. I force myself out of bed, put on a brave face, and try to be a good example. But with them gone five days of the week, I fear I will fall into depression. The silence is too loud, the emptiness too vast. Without them here, it's easier to succumb to the pain, to stay in bed and let the world pass by.

I sit on the edge of my bed, staring at the empty house. The fight feels harder now, but I have to keep pushing through, for them and for myself. It's a new chapter, and I must believe I can handle the challenges ahead, even when it feels impossible.

The room feels heavy with silence. I close my eyes, trying to find some peace, but pain, fear, and shame swim around me. The past months of therapy have been a rollercoaster of emotions—anger, sadness, frustration, shame. Every session feels like I'm unlocking a new piece of the puzzle, a new truth about myself that I've been trying to ignore for years.

Is this how it's supposed to be? In the aftermath of each session, fear creeps in. I'm left alone with my thoughts, wondering if I'm doing the right thing. Then doubt sets in, doubt that I'll ever be able to heal, doubt that I'll ever be able to be whole again.

My mind sweeps even further back, to my childhood and dark memories I kept secret for so long and the decisions I made to escape the pain of that time by moving far away. Leaving my family behind as a teenager was the hardest thing I'd done, but my determination to escape that life and help others in India was stronger.

It hits me now. All the while, I was running away from myself. I blamed myself for first allowing the abuse and then revealing that abuse and causing the breakup of my family. I thought that by dedicating myself fully to my work and charitable endeavours, I could redeem myself.

Tears stream down my face.

My ability in my adult years to protect myself has carried me through some dark and deep traumas, but my therapist told me that I now need to offer space, love, and compassion to the parts I have buried so deep within me that I have forgotten them. I wonder if I only remember selective things, and if so, why?

The question makes me think of a conversation I had with my son during the weekend. I asked Ryan if he has friends he can trust. He told me almost everyone in his class gets along with him, but there was no one he felt comfortable talking to about his problems. I reminded him of a friend he had in primary school, who sat with him when he was crying. The friend told a teacher and his mother about kids who were being mean to Ryan, so he could get the help he needed.

"Do you remember you were crying after a rough day, so I took you for a hot chocolate at Hook and Ladder, and we talked about what happened in school?" I asked him.

He looked down, then back at me again, "I don't remember the crying bit, but I do remember the hot chocolate." Even the kind gesture of his friend was not part of his train of thought anymore.

"So, you just remember the good stuff. That's great," I told him.

Our conversation made me think about how people can choose to *focus* on different things, causing them to *remember* different things. I remember every aspect of certain parts of my childhood; they come back to my mind with intense feelings still attached, but other parts are just a blur. Maybe it's a coping mechanism. It seems my body has retained all those emotions, though, and held them inside for too long.

I want to understand myself better, but I also need to protect myself. If my body, mind, and soul decided that I couldn't handle something and chose to suppress certain memories, maybe it's because they were too painful. It could be the hurt I felt or things I couldn't understand at such a young age. Revisiting them now might help me heal, but it could also bring pain, which makes me cautious. I'm already dealing with pain. Do I want more of it?

To find freedom from this ongoing struggle with invisible-yet-very-real pain, I feel the need to access deeper parts of myself. But I need methods to help me feel safe while doing this, working with my therapist to find patterns (and hopefully, solutions) to my physical condition. I know it's not all in my mind, but I have discovered a link between stress and tension and increased pain levels and fatigue. My mind really does affect my body and general well-being.

After so many years of keeping busy, running from my past and parts of myself, I need to engage in a dialogue of love, kindness, compassion, and care for those hurting parts. I've bottled up so much for so long, stuffing my emotions into an invisible jar and suppressing them to where I now have a hard time accessing them.

This is why I have difficulty showing kindness to myself. It's one area I need to grow in—offering myself compassion, not demanding too much, honouring the strides I make to move forward.

Perhaps healing for me is letting go of things that hold me back or people who drain me with their constant negative attitudes. Perhaps healing is valuing myself for who I am—trusting that the strength, courage, and willpower I possess will see me through. Perhaps healing is learning to live with my condition by adjusting my expectations, giving myself grace and compassion to make mistakes, prioritising self-care, and treating myself with the same kindness and understanding I would give to a dear friend.

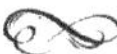

I glance out the window. The rain is coming down in torrents, and the wind is howling, bending the trees. Despite the weather warning, I am cosy and comfortable on my round sofa, snuggled up in pyjamas with my blanket and teddy bears supporting me. A China teacup, filled with warm and aromatic chai, sits on a small table at my side.

As I look outside, I notice an evergreen tree standing tall and unyielding. Its branches sway with the wind, but the tree always returns to its natural state—reaching toward the sky, giving shelter to the birds nesting in its leaves. The birds chirp away, oblivious to the storm raging around them.

The evergreen reminds me of my own struggles, my inner strength, and my faith. Just as the tree stands firm in thc facc of thc storm, so do I. I have been battling an illness for so many long and strenuous months, but I am still here, fighting with courage, faith, perseverance, and grace.

The pain is still excruciating and relentless, and it takes many forms: there is throbbing pain, electric shock pain, burning pain, cutting pain, and stabbing pain. I've learned that resisting the pain only makes it persist. When I embrace it and acknowledge it, it's a way of telling my body I see what it's trying to do for me. My body is a wonderful thing, capable of taking so much, but I need to take care of it.

As I sit here with my laptop, blanket, and tea, I feel grateful for this moment of peace in the midst of the storm. The storm that rages outside my window is a reflection of the storm that life keeps throwing my way. But I am still here. I am still standing. I have not given up, and I won't start now.

Chapter 20

Mobility Scooters and Car Races

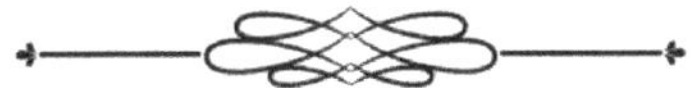

"I don't know how I'm going to make it through the park tomorrow," I say to Anthony as we make our way to the pier in North Dublin. The wind from the sea is biting, and I wrap myself up tightly to block it.

"We can always get a wheelchair for you," Anthony suggests, smiling at me.

I'm not sure if he's joking or serious. "Let's see how I feel tomorrow," I reply, still feeling uncertain.

Later that night, I toss and turn in the lumpy hotel bed. "This bed is terrible," I complain to Anthony, who is awake beside me, also trying to find a comfortable position.

"I know, but we should have said something earlier."

"It's too late now," I say with a sigh.

I didn't sleep well, and now I'm paying the price for it. My back is killing me, and it's hard to move around as we prepare to leave the hotel and head to Tayto Park. I struggle to stay upright, let alone think about walking the whole day. I don't plan to go on any rides at the amusement park. Instead, I'll take care of the bags and jackets and take pictures. Hopefully, my boys will enjoy themselves. But I'm starting to wonder if I will need to ask for a wheelchair before the day is over.

We arrive, and the boys are a whirl of noise and excitement in the back seat as they look out the window at the roller coasters. I listen to their conversation about rides they hope to go on, struggling inwardly. I don't want to spoil the day for them by not keeping up, but I am exhausted after a sleepless night and in a lot of pain. I'm already bundled from head to toe, particularly the head to keep away the wind that often causes intense surges of pain.

Swallow your pride and ask for the wheelchair, my inner voice rings as I get out of the car. It doesn't hurt to find out if they have one.

I tuck jackets into the food bag and ask my boys to carry it. I am only holding my phone and myself, putting one foot in front of the other. It feels great to walk and I know it helps get the blood moving in my body. But after just 200 metres, I feel like I have no more energy to keep going. The mixture of exhaustion, lack of sleep, and two weeks of constant lower back pain is not making it any easier.

"Love, did you ask for the wheelchair?" I ask Anthony as he starts towards us with the wristbands in his hands.

"Oh, sorry, I didn't. Do you still want it?" He looks at me with a doubtful expression, like he's wondering if I am really going to do this.

"Yes, I think I'll need it." I want to get through the day, and if a wheelchair will help, so be it.

Anthony goes back to inquire about it, and we get passed from one person to another. Finally, a customer service lady sees us and says that they only have motorised scooters, which she describes as a mobility aid. A light-hearted staff member jokes as he brings in the scooter, "Don't make donuts with them." He laughs at his own joke, and my husband joins in.

I stare at the motorised scooter with a little basket in the front to carry small things. *I'm going to look like a granny in this.*

My thoughts are echoed by both my boys. "Mom, you look like one of those old people who can't get around." They laugh, and I catch their gaze, giving them both the mom look.

"Please don't joke about it. It's hard enough to need one of these."

"Look, Mom, you can carry the backpack." Collin takes the backpack from his shoulders and places it on the scooter where my foot is resting.

"Well, at least you have one less thing to carry, Collin." He smiles and rushes off to check out the rides.

"How does this work?" I wonder aloud as I look down at small lights showing the batteries are full. To the right, there is a knob with a picture of a turtle on one end and a hare at the other. I assume that's for speed.

Then there are two levers. I press one and start moving forward; I press the other and move backwards. Any time I let go of the lever, the scooter comes to an abrupt stop. *Okay. I can do this.*

While I'm trying to get the hang of the scooter, I am in the dead centre of the entrance. Families are entering the park, staff members are coming and going, and there is a lot happening around me. I start feeling eyes on me. People are looking at me, and I'm sure they are passing judgement. *Yes, I am 38 years old and using a mobility assistive scooter.*

"Keep up, slowpoke," Anthony calls out humorously as I try to manoeuvre the scooter without hitting anything or inviting the stares of passersby. Is it just me or are they staring, wondering why I can't walk? I feel so self-conscious, like I'm being judged for using this scooter.

I can't do this. I feel tears prickling in my eyes. *I don't want to be here. I don't want to be a burden to anyone. I just want to go home.*

But I can't go home, not when my boys are here, not when they are waiting for me to take pictures of them and share in their joy.

"Mom, hurry up! We want to go on the rides!" Collin shouts from a distance.

I take a deep breath and wipe away the tears. I remind myself that I am strong. If anyone has a problem with me using this scooter, it's their problem, not mine.

I push the lever forward, and the scooter picks up speed. I take in the sights and sounds around me, feeling the wind blowing through my hair. It's not so bad, actually.

"Hey, Mom, check out that ride! We're going on that one next!" Collin shouts excitedly, pointing at a roller coaster in the distance.

"Awesome, let's get a picture in front of it!" I say, reaching for my phone. We stop to take the picture, and I feel a small sense of pride.

As I make my way through the park, emotions are all mixed up inside me. I feel relief and gratitude for having the scooter to help me get around. Without it, I would have been confined to a bench, watching my family have fun from a distance. But I can't completely move past my self-consciousness and embarrassment. It's hard to shake the feeling that people are looking at me and judging me for being in a mobility scooter when there is nothing visible that makes it apparent I would need one.

As the day goes on, I slowly begin to relax and enjoy myself more. I take pictures of my husband and boys on the rides and capture their joy and excitement. We share snacks and laughter. I know we are creating memories that will last a lifetime. The mobility scooter is not a symbol of my disability, but a tool that allows me to fully participate in life with those I love.

As we head back to the hotel at the end of the day, I am exhausted but content. As I settle into a new hotel bed, I whisper a silent thank you to myself for accepting help and letting go of my pride. I may have an invisible illness, but I was able to enjoy the day with my family. And that's all that matters.

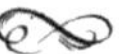

As I sit on my couch watching the Formula 1 Grand Prix on TV, memories flood my mind. I remember the excitement I felt as a child when I first watched the high-speed race. The sound of the engines roaring, the burning rubber, and the adrenaline rush of the drivers filled me with awe.

The laps of the race, which usually range from 50 to 70 depending on the circuit, are a true test of endurance, skill, and strategy. The drivers navigate hairpin turns and straightaways at speeds of up to 220 mph, all while jockeying for position and avoiding collisions with other cars. The tension is palpable in the crowd as the laps count down and the drivers push themselves and their cars to the limit.

I wonder how one of those drivers would feel if suddenly their car started acting up, if it just decided to slow down or stop working all together. That's what it feels like battling an illness that has forced me to slow down. My body, once a powerhouse, is now weak and vulnerable. I can sense the disconnect between my mind—which is still as sharp and active as ever—and my body that no longer cooperates as it used to.

It's a daily struggle to find a balance between pushing myself enough to avoid stagnation and not overexerting myself. I have the worst triad for this kind of illness; I am a Type A personality, a perfectionist, and competitive. I feel like a damaged Ferrari, still holding on to memories of power, speed, and invincibility but unable to compete due to a severe accident. My engine, once amazing, still thinks it can run laps and come in first, but my chassis won't cooperate.

The internal battle between my brain and my body rages. I know what I was once capable of, and I can see the racetrack in my mind. I long to be back in the race, to feel the rush of speed and adrenaline once again, but those days are gone, perhaps for good. I need to find a way to be happy and fulfilled while managing my pain and subsequent weight gain.

I must accept where I am *now* and focus on what I can do. I need to be kind to myself and remember that I am doing the best I can. Perhaps one day, I will find a way to return to the Grand Prix, but for now I must focus on the race within myself.

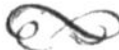

It is November 2021, and three years have slipped away, silently marking the passage of time since the onset of my illness. I hesitate to call it an "anniversary" because there's nothing to celebrate.

The past few days have forced me to confront the significance of that date three years ago. The cold of winter has intensified my pain, making each day a struggle. I wake to find the discomfort sharper, with the chill in the air seeping into my bones, amplifying the ache. Simple tasks become monumental challenges, and the shorter, grey days add to the heaviness I feel.

Three years ago, I was working in my office, feeling invincible and climbing the career ladder with confidence. My life seemed perfectly on track, full of promise and success. I was blissfully unaware of the swirling storm that lay ahead: chronic pain and an invisible illness that would soon become my daily reality.

Although three long years have elapsed, I sense that I am still at the beginning of my personal journey. It's a daunting thought. The process of reprogramming myself is not an overnight endeavour, particularly when I find myself deeply entrenched in old patterns of ploughing through obstacles instead of sitting with the discomfort and seeing what it's trying to teach me.

It is time to recalibrate, to create space and grant myself time for introspection, allowing my gaze to turn inward. It's time to open myself up and resist the instinct to close off from the pain, the hurt, and the traumas that have marked my journey thus far.

It's time for a deeper dive into the core of my being—confronting my fears head-on and looking them in the eye with love and compassion. This expedition into the uncharted territories of my life demands a reassessment of the beliefs, thoughts, and stories I have clung to.

Today, I have a meeting with my therapist, our first in three weeks due to her absence for holidays and training. One of the things she encouraged me to do during the break was to examine whether I am prepared to confront the issues we need to work through together.

I am preparing myself to accept the inevitability of time. Yes, time—the word I once loathed to hear. In the past, this word provoked frustration, anger, and impatience whenever doctors or therapists spoke of it.

Waiting has never been my strong suit. I wanted everything instantaneously, now! Yet here I find myself far from where I had hoped to be, unsure when this hourglass will finally turn. As the grains of sand trickle down, each one an indication of the slow passage of time, I look up and realise the considerable amount of sand that must fall before I can turn it again.

I am trapped within the confines of time, and I must make peace with that in order to move forward. Otherwise, I sense my body will suffer even greater consequences. So, it is about taking time—making time—for myself. It's about embracing self-love, tenderness, and compassion for the gradual progress I am making.

Here is what I will rejoice in now: that I can now engage in ten minutes of exercise such as walking and doing slow movements in the pool, that I can still drive a vehicle, even if my parking skills and spatial awareness leave much to be desired. I find comfort in the freedom of mobility I still possess even if it is nothing like I had in the past.

In my moments of repose, I no longer subject myself to harsh self-judgement. I can enjoy podcasts and leisurely scroll through Facebook from the comfort of my bed. I take pleasure in the sunlight that spills through my window, and I lately have been carving out time for writing.

These may seem like trivial victories, but they are the consistent, incremental steps I am taking. They are the small but significant movements that will eventually alter my course entirely. In realising this, I feel a weight lift from my shoulders, buoyed by the knowledge that I am doing all I can to progress, no matter how slowly.

I open my journal and begin to write my hopes for the days ahead, for this turn of the hourglass:

May this inward journey illuminate the powerful soul that resides within me. May it grant me the strength to conquer my fears, replacing them with confidence and courage, knowing that what I am doing is the very best for myself. May healing emerge from within, permeating every aspect of my existence.

As I download this new program, may it reveal to me the extraordinary, resilient, and indomitable person I am and have always been. May I discover the capacity for self-compassion, embracing the mistakes and perceived failures that have marked my path. And above all, may this journey within bestow upon me the fortitude to continue battling and facing my physical pain with grace and love.

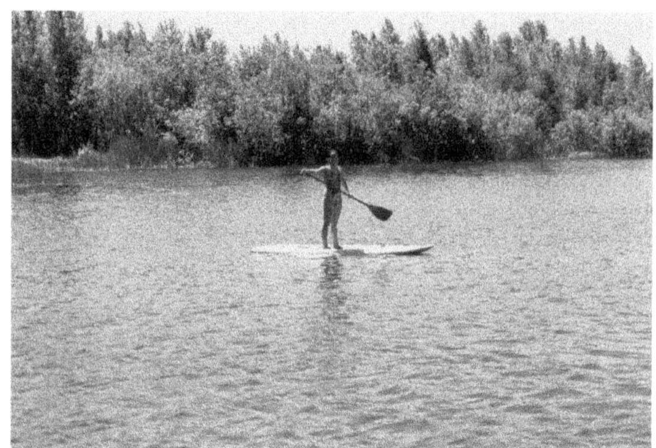

Duluth - Minnesota - USA

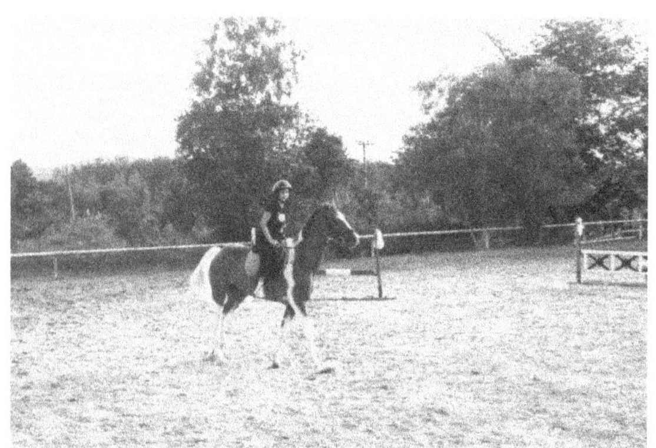

Rayong - Thailand

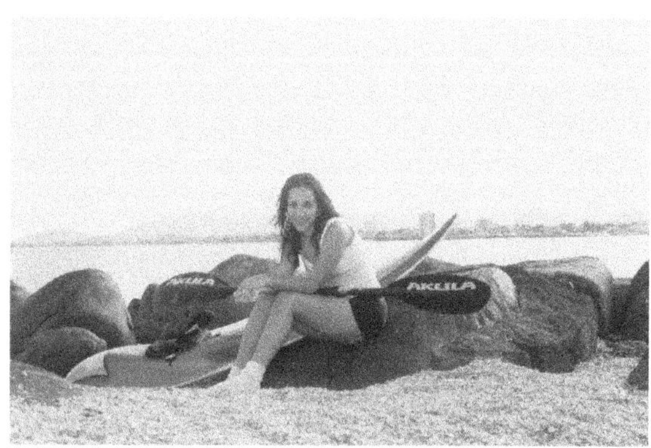

Barra Velha - SC - Brazil

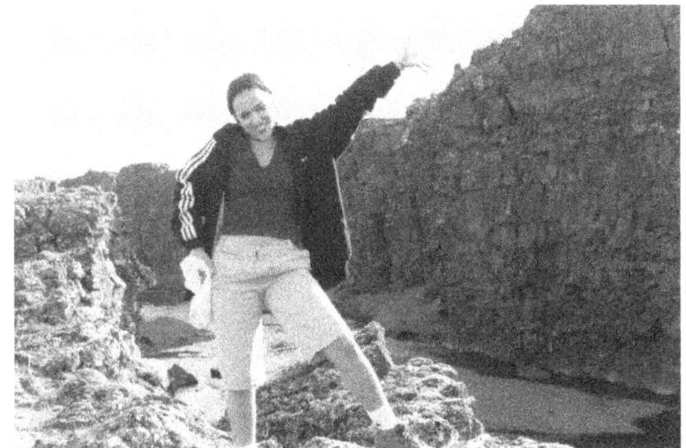

Þingvellir National Park - Iceland

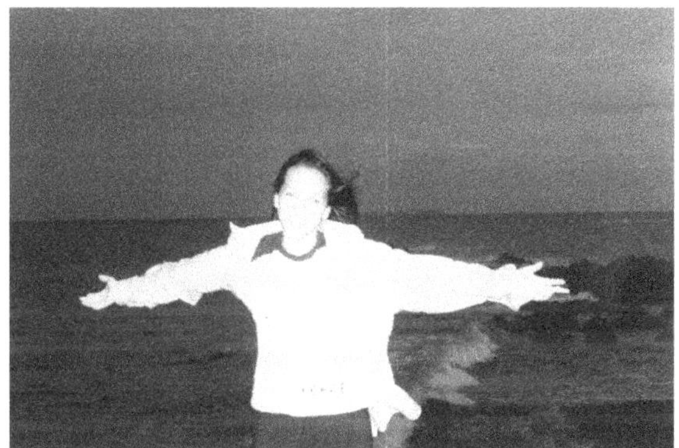

Penang - Malaysia

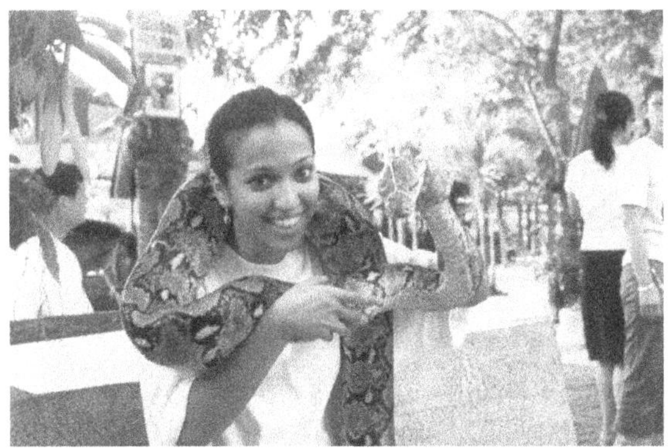

Bangkok - Thailand

Part 4: What Healing Means

"It takes courage to be the real you, and it's also the only path you'll ever find to true freedom. It takes risk to be the real you, and it's also the only possibility of experiencing true purpose. It takes vulnerability to be the real you, and it's also the only place you'll experience true love. Showing up in this world as ALL of who you are tastes like freedom."

– **Jamie Kern Lima,** *Worthy: How to Believe You Are Enough and Transform Your Life*

Chapter 21

Achievable Goals

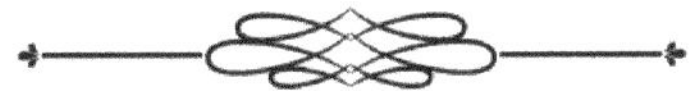

It's January 3rd, 2022. I always get excited about the possibilities of a new year and set ambitious goals for myself. I see the new year as an opportunity to assess my life and plan to do better. Always better. But the problem is, I tend to overstretch and end up fizzling out. I've learned this about myself over the years, but it's been especially difficult since my health has been hijacked.

Last year, I stripped back my goals to focus on my health, but I'm still hesitant to set any new ones this year. I know I should be focusing on getting better, but I want something measurable, something that feels like a tangible achievement. Focusing on my health means accepting small, incremental changes, like being able to go for a 10-minute walk or breathe through surges of pain. But these accomplishments feel insignificant, too small to really celebrate. It's hard not to fall into depression when my goals don't align with my expectations.

I turn 40 this year, and I had a very different vision of what my life would look like by now. I wanted to have a huge party, surrounded by all my friends from around the world. Dancing and celebrating are what I love most, and my birthday is the one time of year where I don't feel guilty about putting myself first. But in my fourth year of dealing with this invisible illness, the thought of turning 40 discourages me.

The resistance within me is still strong. I constantly wrestle with who I was and who I think I should be by now. I need to find solid ground to stabilise myself on. I want to focus on something to celebrate, but my expectations are hard to downplay. I'd love to be a millionaire, even though I know an accomplishment like that is not easy and takes a lot of energy, stamina, and drive to achieve. Right now, I need to accept my reality and set goals that are achievable in my current state.

Dialogue with my therapist helps me gain clarity. She reminds me that slow and steady progress wins the race. It's important to focus on my health and take small steps towards progress, she says. Yes, I should be proud of every breath I take, every bit of energy I muster, and every moment of pain I endure without letting it consume me. These small steps are significant achievements, and they are a proof of my resilience.

I may not be able to measure my health in external ways like I can with a language or career goal, but I can measure it within myself. I feel the changes, no matter how small they may seem. And that's something to celebrate.

My therapist also reminds me that it's okay to celebrate myself, even if it's not my birthday. Maybe that should be a new year goal: make time for myself and do things that bring me joy.

As I reflect on my journey to acceptance, I realise that my illness has taught me to appreciate the little things in life. Did it really take trigeminal neuralgia to make me finally stop and smell the roses, to slow down, be more mindful, and take care of myself?

While I may not be where I thought I would be at this point in my life, I jot down some of the lessons I've learned over the past few years, and I realize that I am truly grateful.

This year, I will set goals, but in keeping with the person I am now:

I will focus on my health and celebrate minor achievements.

I will plan a small birthday party with my loved ones, to remind myself that it's okay to put myself first and celebrate who I am!

Sometimes the universe has a way of showing us that our adjusted expectations can lead to unexpected magic. While I have let go of my dreams of a grand fortieth celebration, my loved ones have other plans. They understand something I am still learning—that celebrating doesn't have to be diminished just because it looks different than we imagined.

And celebrate we do! My fortieth birthday turns out to be nothing like my original vision, yet somehow it becomes everything I need it to be. My husband and cousins transform a private room in an upscale venue into a magical space, with metallic golden and black balloon arches creating an ethereal entrance. Walking through floor-length golden shimmer curtains feels like stepping into another world—one where chronic illness doesn't define the boundaries of joy.

My husband insisted I rest beforehand, arranging for a friend to accompany me to the party, and now I understand why. Every detail speaks of love: black-clothed tables adorned with golden balloons and sparkles, comfortable sofas creating intimate spaces for conversation, and a stunning three-tier chocolate cake featuring my favourites—Ferrero Rocher and Raffaello—surrounded by scattered chocolates that gleam like precious stones under the lights.

Latin music flows through the speakers, and though I can't dance as much as I once did, the rhythm still moves my soul. Having exactly forty people present—friends who have driven from Dublin, Cork, and Galway, neighbours who have become family, and loved ones from Limerick—feels like a perfect synchronicity. As we play games and share laughter, I find myself fully present in each moment, my pain taking a backseat to the joy surrounding me. The party proves what my heart has been trying to tell me all along: that celebration doesn't require grand gestures or perfect health, just the courage to show up and let yourself be seen and loved.

My cup of joy isn't just full—it's overflowing with gratitude for this beautiful reminder that life's sweetest moments often come when we learn to celebrate exactly where we are.

Chapter 22

THERAPIES

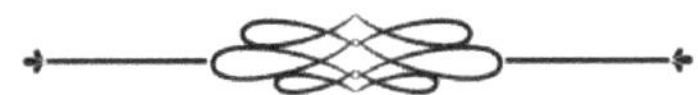

As I walk into my physiotherapist's room, a familiar tension builds up in my neck, signalling a migraine. My face feels numb, and the left eye socket is sore as if someone punched me. My physio quickly picks up on my discomfort, and she suggests different positions for me to relax in. I try lying face down, but it's impossible. I try lying on my left side, but half a minute later I start shifting, looking for a position that won't hurt.

"Maybe we should try sitting on a chair," she suggests, "and leaning your upper body forward on the bed with a pillow to prop you up so I can work on your neck and back."

I try it, but the pressure in my head remains, so she suggests just sitting in the chair, closing my eyes, and working from there. It helps; there's no pressure on my head, and I can finally relax into her hands. With each gentle move, she kneads tense muscles, bringing circulation back to my neck.

As she works, she speaks softly about my thoughts, and I can feel her steady hands calming me. "Michele, I feel that the breathing techniques don't work for you as much as we hoped," she says. "Your mind overthinks, and you over-analyse things. All that tension causes the body to create stress chemicals, making it overactive. You need to find out what will help you not take on so much stress because it's physically hurting you."

I know she's right, but it's hard to let go of my natural tendency to fix things. I can feel people deeply and understand them in a profound way because I care about them. But the downside is that I take on their problems, mulling them over and looking for ways to solve them. My physio and I connect over this, as she's mentioned a similar tendency in wanting to help others.

"Learning to let people help themselves is vital," she told me in a previous session.

Today, she reminds me of how we can feed our thoughts. "Picture someone going for a scan," she says. "Your mind creates a scenario, and your body feels it as if it's a real threat." I can relate; my mom is going for a scan this week, and I feel the added stress and tension, almost as if it's me having the scan.

"Focus on things that bring you joy, Michele. Remember, you need to take care of yourself instead of trying to control everything and everyone around you."

Controlling the outcome has always been my way of making the world feel safe; this is how I want it to be, but it's not how the world works. It's hard to admit that, even to myself.

"You're right. I need to work on letting go of control, stop trying to fix everything and everyone, and learn to be okay with things being in flux."

My physiotherapist nods. "It's not easy, but it's important. It's like dancing; you have to let go of control and trust the flow." Her words hit home. I used to dance—a long time ago. I wonder if I've forgotten how.

It will be a slow journey toward an approach of acceptance rather than control, but I'm willing to take the first steps toward finding a new way of being.

Sitting on my couch, journal in hand, I reflect on the realization that my desire to control and plan ahead is a coping mechanism, a way to mitigate what could go wrong and pre-empt it. This rigidity has made it hard for me to enjoy life and find pleasure in the small things.

Growing up, I refused to follow the crowd. I never got tattoos, dyed my hair, or pierced my nose just because everyone else was doing it. Now my once gorgeous black hair is getting more and more white strands. My son even commented that my hair is beginning to look like the moon. It's making me reconsider my stance on things like using hair dye.

Maybe it's time to let go of my stubbornness. Rigidity is not serving me on this journey toward healing, and I need to free myself from the shackles of wanting to control it all.

Free Michele! That's what my physiotherapist told me. But how? Maybe by allowing myself to believe things *can* be different. That I can listen to a new voice, a new tune, and have fun in the process. That I can accept the things I cannot change and allow things to be just as they are.

If I can let the wind take me and trust my instincts to carry me, part of me knows that I can find health, healing, bonding, laughter, and fun. Another part of me still wants to take control of it all to protect myself and others from frightening possibilities.

I am blessed to have a family that loves and supports me, but I need to make healthy space for myself, too. I want to enjoy the small things, like sunsets and baths in Epson salts. I want to listen to my body more and help my mind rest and not be consumed by emotions. I want to let go and let others sort themselves out.

I cannot control the outcome, but I can control the next thought I have, as Dr. Caroline Leaf so aptly explains in the NeuroCycle five-step program. I can make this new way of thinking a central part of who I am. It will take time, but I know that it will be worth it.

So, I write these words down, telling myself I will return to them often.

I will allow myself to be free, to find pleasure in the small things, and to let go of control.

Free Michele! Let's do this!

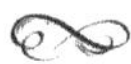

I enter the room, and the scent of lavender and vanilla envelops me, an invitation to calm my nerves. The room is dimly lit with flickering candlelight, offering a tranquil ambiance. In the centre of the room, a massage bed draped with a colourful patterned sarong awaits me. The sarong's silky texture feels cool to the touch.

On one side of the room, three Tibetan bowls are arranged, each bowl a different size. The largest bowl is as big as a basketball, while the smallest is the size of a grapefruit. The bowls are beautifully decorated with etched designs. It is my first experience in sound therapy. My massage therapist is learning sound therapy and offered me this free experience.

Angel figurines and dream catchers hang on the walls, and I wonder if it's all a little woo-woo. I remind myself to immerse into the experience without taking it apart or questioning how effective all these things really can be.

As I lie down on the massage bed, the therapist invites me to lie on my back and close my eyes. She moves around me and begins tapping the bowls, and their soft, metallic hum fills the air. The vibrations ripple through my body. The sound is both ethereal and grounding.

The bowls continue to hum, and their sound grows louder and more intense. Each bowl makes a unique sound, yet they work in perfect harmony. I feel the vibrations in every cell of my body. It's like a dance between my body and the sound, each movement in perfect sync with the other.

I surrender myself to the sensation, letting myself be present with the vibration, with the rhythm, with the dance as it flows through my very core, and it energises me. I can't explain why or how, but I feel relaxed, at peace, and surrendered.

As the session ends, I feel renewed and rejuvenated. The practice, once unfamiliar, now feels like a sanctuary, a space for healing and restoration. The Tibetan bowls have worked their magic, and I am grateful for this moment of peace and stillness.

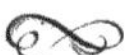

In my relentless quest for pain relief, I've explored a plethora of treatments, leaving no stone unturned. I rest on my back on a cozy bed, in the middle of yet another acupuncture session. Needles, despite being my sworn enemies, are strategically placed on my forehead, hands, and various points on my legs and feet. It's an odd paradox, but here I am, engaging in conversation with a doctor who has traded the conventional for the ancient, delving into the realms of Eastern medicine, particularly acupuncture.

As I lie here, trying to embrace the discomfort, the doctor paints a picture of how these tiny needles will act as architects of a reset, rebalance, and rediscovery of equilibrium within my body.

"Just breathe, Michele. You'll be alright." The doctor's reassurance tempers the prickling sensation. Each needle comes with its own backstory, he explains gently, as if I'm being guided through an intricate map of my own healing.

Once the needles are in place, the doctor exits, leaving me in the company of soft melodies. The soundtrack, mimicking the soothing sound of a waterfall, wraps around me, inviting my body to let go and relax. By the third session, I experience a tangible release of tension and stress.

Acupuncture, once an unexpected ally, is now a stalwart companion, a tool I reach for when the balloon of anxiety threatens to burst. Calming my body and mind, it empowers me to confront pain with resilience and a sense of tranquillity. I am grateful for this unconventional form of therapy, a cornerstone in my arsenal against chronic pain.

The journey then takes a turn toward the chiropractor's office—a pivotal chapter in my ongoing saga. After scouring through recommendations, I embark on a journey to Cork, enduring a 1½-hour drive from Limerick each way. The chiropractor there, armed with extensive knowledge of neurological conditions, guides me through 25 sessions, each crack of the spine a signal of release. Yet, the gruelling commute forces me to rethink my strategy. I need a chiropractor closer to home.

After more research, I finally find one, and under the care of this local chiropractor, I undergo adjustments twice a month. The chiropractor's method is distinct, beginning with me standing, eyes locked on a picture hanging on the wall. Different pressure points on my back become the focus, each touch a diagnostic exploration into balance, imbalance, sensitivity, and pain. The subsequent adjustments—be it a subtle repositioning or a deliberate stretch—form a choreography to align my body. It's a routine that seamlessly integrates into my pain management strategy, providing a crucial piece to the puzzle.

My journey continues through this vast landscape of alternative treatments—a diverse array suggested by well-meaning friends. Healers, acupressure, mediums, sleep psychologists, hypnosis, the Alexander technique, naturopaths, Bowen therapy, dietary shifts, increased vitamin and mineral intake, heat therapy, and even the uncomfortable invigoration of cold showers—all these holistic therapies help in one way or another.

Daily movement also remains a key element in my daily routine; however, I still have not found any one of these methods a key to complete healing. These tools become companions in my ongoing battle against chronic pain.

Chapter 23

Finding the Beat

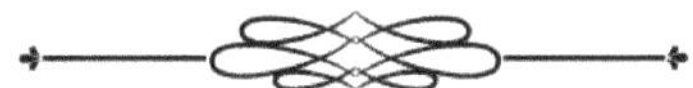

I sit on the couch in my living room, staring blankly at the wall in front of me. My mother is visiting from Brazil. Always eager to help me through my struggles, she is shuffling around the room, tidying up. She pauses to glance over at me, and seeing me still deep in thought, she turns to face me.

"Have you been listening to any music lately?" she asks, her voice tinged with concern.

I shake my head slowly. "No, I don't really feel like it right now."

My mother frowns and comes over to sit next to me on the couch. "That's no good, *filha*. You know how much music can help lift your spirits. Come on, let's listen to some together."

I smile a little at her eagerness. She's always been a big believer in the healing power of music, and as a Brazilian, it's practically in her blood.

She takes out her phone and begins scrolling through her playlist. "How about this one?" She holds up her phone. "It's a classic samba, just the thing to get you moving."

I shake my head again. "I don't think I'm up for dancing right now, Mom."

She scoffs playfully. "Nonsense! You used to love dancing. Come on, let's at least try."

Before I can protest further, she's already up and pulling me to my feet. She hits play on her phone, and the music starts. The beat is infectious, and before I know it, my feet are tapping along.

My mother begins to move, swaying her hips in time with the music. "Come on, *filha*, let yourself feel it!"

I start out slowly, but the rhythm of the music pulls me in. As I move my body, my feet find the beat on their own.

"That's it!" my mother exclaims, clapping her hands. "You've still got it, *filha*!"

We dance to two more songs, my mother twirling me around the room and laughing. I can feel myself starting to loosen up, the constant weight of my current state beginning to lift just a little.

As we dance, my mother starts to hum along with the music. Her voice is rich and warm. I realise how much I've missed hearing her sing. It's one of the things I love most about her, the way she can make even the simplest melody sound beautiful.

We dance until we're both out of breath. My mother looks over at me, her eyes shining with joy.

"You see?" she says, beaming. "Music is good for the soul. You need to get back to dancing to help heal yourself."

I can't help but smile back at her, feeling lighter than before, at least a little. Maybe she's right. Maybe music is just what I need right now. And who knows? Maybe dancing again will expedite my healing.

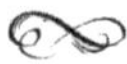

The following Thursday, my mom sits on the couch, phone in hand. The room is immaculate, each surface polished to a shine. She looks over at me. "There has to be a place where we can dance to Latin music." She starts scrolling on her phone and, after a few moments, tilts the screen toward me. "Look at this one."

I glance at the webpage; it's a hall that hosts Latin dance nights once a week.

"This could be perfect," she continues. "Let's call Clara. It'll be a great way for us to get out of the house and have some fun together."

She dials my eldest sister. "Clara, I found this place that has Latin dancing tonight. It would be wonderful for all of us to go. Can you come pick us up? It'll be a nice change of pace."

My mom's face is alight with anticipation as she listens to my sister's response. A minute later, she ends the call and looks at me, her eyes twinkling. "She agreed. We're going dancing."

That evening, my sister drives us to the hall. The air is crisp with the promise of warmer days, and I feel a mix of excitement and apprehension. As we step inside, the vibrant beats of Latin music fill the room. I know these beats. It has been too long since I danced to them.

I position myself at the back of the room, hoping to blend into the background during the warm-up session. Although my view of the instructor is limited, I watch the dancers around me. The warm-up ends, and the instructor instructs us to form a circle and find a partner. Tonight, she explains, we're diving into bachata, a dance that exudes passion and connection.

The music begins, and its sultry melody instantly transports me back to Latin America. The rhythms stir something deep within me, awakening memories and a sense of belonging I have not felt in years.

The instructor, Caoimhe, points at me, singling me out from the circle. Embarrassment and anticipation wash over me as all the dancers turn in my direction.

Reluctantly, I make my way to the centre of the dance floor, standing face to face with Caoimhe. Her touch on my shoulder grounds me as our hands interlock, creating a connection that transcends words. She explains the next move, her voice carrying across the room, and the DJ cues the song.

My body tenses, but Caoimhe senses my unease. "Relax," she whispers. "I've got you. Let go and trust."

I try to anticipate the next move, but the instructor softly says, "Just be in the moment. Let go and feel the music. Allow me to lead you."

As I dance, tension lingers within me. My control-freak nature resists the vulnerability of surrender. Every instinct compels me to take the lead, to anticipate the next move, to cling to the illusion of control.

Yet Caoimhe, with her gentle strength, persists. She somehow recognizes the battle raging within. Her touch on my shoulder becomes firmer, her voice more resolute. "Release the need for control," she urges, her words cutting through the music. "Trust me. Trust the dance."

Frustration washes over me, a desperate longing to break free from the constraints of my own mind. I want to surrender, to let go, but fear holds me captive. Fear of making mistakes, of losing myself in the unknown, of relinquishing control to another's lead.

Caoimhe's eyes meet mine, their intensity piercing through my defences. "You can do this," she reassures me. "Embrace the tension, the struggle, the vulnerability. It's all part of the dance."

With every beat, I feel the battle within me intensify. It's a tug-of-war between control and surrender, fear and trust. The dance becomes a microcosm of my own life, a mirror reflecting my struggle to navigate the uncertainties that accompany my illness.

As the song reaches its crescendo, something inside me shifts. A flicker of acceptance ignites. I realise that control, though comforting, can also be suffocating. It holds me back, preventing me from fully experiencing the beauty and spontaneity of life.

In a moment of clarity, I loosen my grip, releasing the tension in my muscles and allowing the music to guide my moves. I close my eyes and surrender to the dance. We start with two simple steps, moving as one. Caoimhe's touch guides me, her lead carrying me effortlessly across the floor. With each movement, she invites me to release my need for control, to let the music flow through me and dictate my steps.

As I accept Caoimhe's guidance, I stumble occasionally, my body resisting the unfamiliar steps. But instead of frustration, I feel myself relaxing. A smile graces my face. In letting go, in relinquishing control, I find myself in the embrace of freedom. The dance becomes a language of trust and surrender.

This dialog is new for me, but I want more of it. I want to learn to let go of control and allow the rhythm to take me, a bliss in which, for a split second, I don't feel the pain in my physical body, only an unexplainable burst of energy and joy.

Chapter 24

Dancing Through Pain

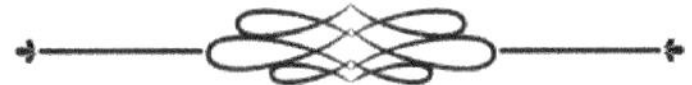

I wake up feeling burdened by pain and exhaustion. Getting out of bed is a struggle, let alone getting the household running smoothly and encouraging my boys to do something productive. Perhaps it's hard for them to find the motivation to do anything when they see me constantly returning to bed.

From my bed, I schedule their annual doctor's appointment for next week. As I hang up the phone, Ryan enters the room.

"Mom, are they still taking kids for the Cadet program with the Order of Malta?" he asks quietly.

"Yes, they are," I reply, sensing his interest. "It's a great opportunity. You'll learn about first aid and emergency services and get to help people."

He nods nonchalantly, but I see the hint of excitement in his eyes. "I guess I can try it out, since I can't do scouts anymore with my new school schedule."

I smile. "I'm proud of you for wanting to explore new things, Ryan. This sounds like a perfect fit."

Ryan leaves the room, and a wave of contentment washes through me. Each time I gather enough energy to get up, it quickly fades away, sending me back to bed, but moments like these make it worthwhile, when I feel I am helping my kids even in small ways.

I open the app Insight Timer and put on a meditation session guided by a woman's calming voice. Her words are uplifting, and I'd love to lie down and listen to this all day, but I need to get up eventually. I have a visitor coming over later.

I decide to play music on Spotify to inspire me. Scrolling, I select the playlist titled *Música brasileira para relaxar* (relaxing Brazilian music). As the lyrics begin and the melodies envelop me, I am instantly transported to another realm.

The first song is an old classic by Tom Jobim, and it brings a smile to my face and warmth to my soul. When did I forget that music holds the key to my emotions, energy, and connection? How did I lose touch with this amazing thing that allows me to express feelings I didn't even know existed?

That first tune carries me out of bed and to the shower. As I step out of the shower, still riding the wave of the melodies, I find myself doing a few small "samba" steps in the bathroom. My feet glide effortlessly over the fluffy green mat by the shower stall. I catch a glimpse of myself in the mirror and delight in my radiant reflection.

The tunes and impromptu samba dance bring back memories of my youth, participating in dancing competitions and celebrating São João, where we would dance to folk songs and have an absolute blast. Music and dance are inseparable companions, especially for a Brazilian. They infuse me with a surge of energy I have not felt in so long!

I keep the songs playing, grab some food for myself, and then relax enough to allow my boys to do whatever they please—they are engrossed in their phones and Xbox, as is typical for teenagers. And you know what? For a change, that's perfectly fine with me.

Although I don't have the energy or desire to bake as I had originally planned, I return to my writing. Whether I'm expressing how I'm feeling, sharing what's happening, or explaining how I'm coping—it's all important. Music allows me to connect with myself, particularly my younger, more playful self.

I wonder if it's just me that feels like this. Or does it happen to all of us? That part of us we might shy away from—the goofy or even the sexy side—lies in wait, yearning for good music to bring it to the surface. Perhaps it's that music liberates us. I know it liberates me. When I listen to upbeat tunes, I feel free from rigidity and constraints.

This morning, the music calls forth carefree memories. The rhythm-infused songs, filled with spice and flavour, transport me to unknown inner spaces as well—places I have yet to explore. Something about music awakens dormant aspects of my being, enabling me to connect, become present, and truly be.

As I tap out the beat with the pen in my hand, I look up from my notebook and notice my little "desert rose," which I've been diligently trying to revive. A tiny new leaf is sprouting. I've provided my little flower with an infrared light, serving as sunlight when the skies are perpetually grey and rainy, but it was touch and go for a while. I'm thrilled by this progress.

Music has reconnected me with myself once again. It helps me feel rooted in my origins and reminds me of the need for colour, nature, and soothing sounds that comfort, heal, and restore me.

I respond to this need by bringing more plants and flowers into my home. After an impromptu visit to a garden nursery, I acquire three lush green plants and six small flowers and succulents. I place them throughout the house. It's delightful to descend the stairs each day and be greeted by their verdant presence. There's a purple flower with delicate white petals, green Ficus plants adorned with touches of white on their leaves, a deep purple succulent, and an aloe vera-like plant gracing my dining room.

They are scattered throughout the ground floor, while my precious "Rosa do deserto" (desert rose) resides in my bedroom. I constantly check on her, tending to her needs, speaking words of encouragement, rooting for her.

It feels completely natural that my rediscovery of music has connected me with life in this way—has tethered me to the core of who I am. I could proclaim my Irish identity due to the passport I hold, but the truth is, I am Brazilian. I was born and raised there. Those roots, those ties, are the blood that still flows through my veins, and it's crucial for me to honour that part of my being.

There are two sides to me—the peaceful side and the warrior. This balance has been disrupted within me for some time, but by rediscovering my roots, by rediscovering my voice—whether through writing or in life—I can stand on both feet and find equilibrium.

Maybe it's about time to resurrect the part that enjoys music and dance—which embody movement and vitality! It's the healing energy I need to tap into more deeply.

Playing music at home is an experience I'm no longer accustomed to. I've grown fond of silence, and while it has its merits, I realize it also contributed to my rapid decline into sadness and despondency when my invisible illness first hit. But when I listen to good, upbeat songs—especially the Brazilian melodies that resonate with me—they evoke wonderful memories and reawaken a dormant part of my soul.

I want to remain awake. I want to revel in the movements, lyrics, melodies, and beats that carry me away. I want to view life with passion—not through the lens of drowning in my own sadness and ailments, not as someone who has suffered and shut out the world as a result.

I long to be the person who finds joy in awkward conversations, embraces the rhythm of music, and feels the electric current surging through my veins when I hear an upbeat song! If that's where my healing lies, if it where I can reconnect with myself, restore my inner strength, and achieve a new state of mind, body, and spirit—I want to dance even when I am uncertain about the steps and have to relinquish control.

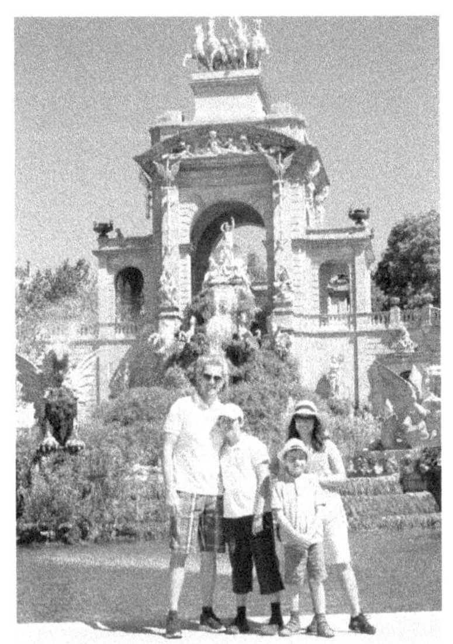

The Parc de la Ciutadella - Barcelona - Spain

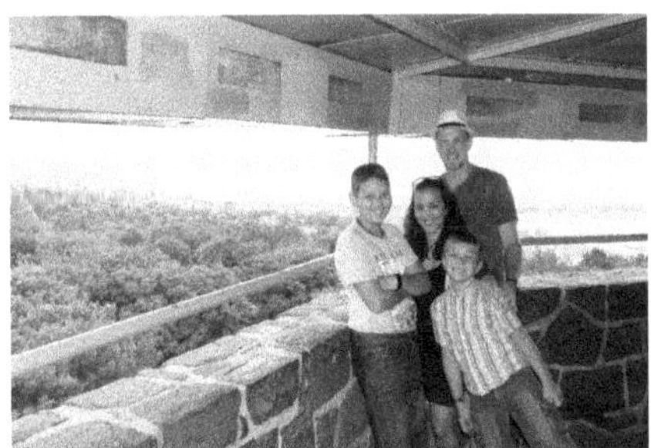

Enger Park Tower - Duluth - Minnesota - USA

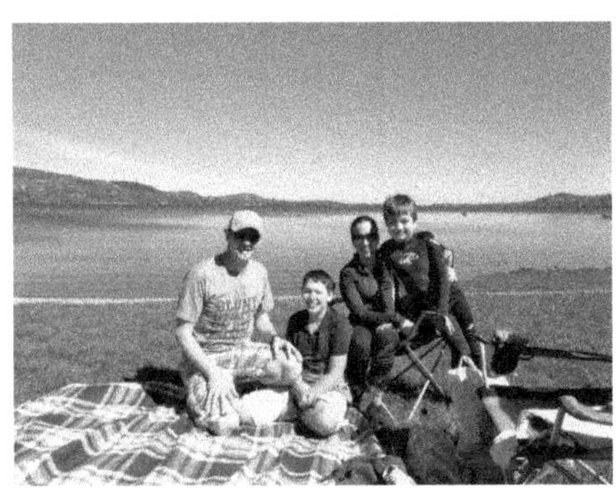

Killaloe - Co. Clare - Ireland

Part 5: Learning to Flow and Grow

"My mission in life is not merely to survive, but to thrive; and to
do so with some passion, some compassion,
some humor, and some style."
– **Maya Angelou**

Chapter 25

Letting Go & Opening Up

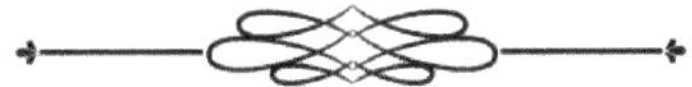

I am making progress, slowly but steadily. During a recent session with my psychologist, I mustered the courage to share the small steps I've taken to protect myself from overextending. I've been setting boundaries with my sibling and stepping away from over-caring for my extended family.

While it feels selfish, I've come to realise that letting those I love care for themselves might actually foster their personal growth. It's like making a nest uncomfortable to keep eaglets from remaining chicks, encouraging them to become eagles that gracefully soar high in the sky.

Countless analogies flood my mind, but the truth remains—I need to prioritise my own well-being, just as the safety instructions on an airplane instruct you to put on your own oxygen mask before assisting others. This image resonates deeply with me, although my instinct has always been to help everyone else before tending to myself.

This, to me, signifies progress.

Apart from that, I sense that I've reached a pivotal point in my therapy where I can open up even further. I recently divulged to my psychologist the identity of the person responsible for my childhood sexual abuse. However, a recent change in legislation regarding reporting abuse has complicated matters. Now that I've confided in her about my experiences, she's obligated to write a report and send it to the child agency in Brazil, my home country.

They will subsequently reach out to me, seeking additional details which I can choose to provide or withhold. They also have the power to involve the authorities, and if they decide to do so, the police in Brazil may be contacted.

Nevertheless, since I haven't disclosed specific names or locations, there isn't much they can act upon.

This is immensely frustrating. Finally, I mustered the strength to reveal my long-held secret, only to discover that the reason I've kept it all buried for years was that I wanted nothing to come of it. I wanted to leave it in the past, a firmly closed chapter in my life. While I strive to heal myself and learn from what happened, I don't want my stepfather to face any repercussions. In my eyes, he has already paid a heavy price for his actions.

I feel apprehensive. I find myself restrained, unable to fully open up. I must meticulously choose my words, ensuring they reveal no identifying information. Yet, by merely stating it was my stepfather, it doesn't take a genius to figure out his identity. I already feel trapped in this situation.

While I can continue my inner work in a roundabout way, the heart of the matter will remain an impasse. I don't want to delve into a legal ordeal. All I seek is my own healing journey. Just hearing my psychologist acknowledge that I wasn't at fault and allowing my wounded inner child to hear those words brought me to tears.

For years, I carried the weight of guilt over my mom's separation from my stepfather and the turmoil my family endured—especially my younger siblings—because of me. I believed that I single-handedly caused my parents to split and set off a never-ending cycle of hardship. Every time I visited, I tried anything I could to help them—buying groceries, showering them with gifts, saving every penny I could—to alleviate my guilt over the hardships they endured because I told the truth about what I had suffered.

It was an immense burden that haunted me. When my stepfather and mother reconciled and my mother became pregnant again, I knew those events were beyond my influence; however, that scared little girl within me had no one to blame but herself. And so, I internalised it all, locking it away.

During my teenage years, I developed a habit of scratching myself—an attempt to regulate the overwhelming surge of emotions I struggled to handle. Everything felt muddled, too much to bear, and finding a new life in a faraway place like India seemed like the best choice.

It has taken me two years to reach this point in my counselling and therapy, only to encounter this barrier that has suddenly appeared. How can I receive the help I need when legal regulations make it nearly impossible to reveal my secrets? I don't want to involve authorities or deal with the hassle and emotional toll that would come with it.

If I continue unearthing long-buried memories, there may be consequences I'm not prepared to face. For now, putting my thoughts on paper provides an outlet—a way to voice my concerns and prevent them from festering. I refuse to allow them to take root in my body. That's the last thing I want.

Deep breaths, Michele...

Inhale...

Exhale...

Inhale peace...

Exhale tension...

Inhale love...

Exhale worries...

You are strong, you are loved, you are more than capable. You are light, radiating peace, and embodying courage.

Chapter 26

Finding Community

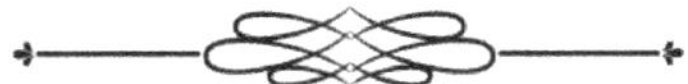

I travel to the Algarve, in Portugal, to attend a dance conference where bachata, salsa, zouk, and kizomba intertwine. Among them, kizomba holds a unique allure for me. Its unhurried pace, its attunement to the moment, is a therapy in itself.

Exhaustion weighs heavily on me from the long flight. It is 11 pm by the time I enter the apartment I will be staying in. My room is on the ground floor, adjacent to the front door. Each time the front door opens, the noise resounds through the halls. And when it slams shut, it reverberates with a force that rattles my bones.

I'm unaccustomed to such disturbances. Sleep eludes me. People come and go throughout the night. Sleeping away from my own bed is already challenging, but the constant ebb and flow of visitors jerks me awake time and again.

Morning arrives, and in addition to the constant coming and going, construction work begins in the apartment right above me. The pound of a hammer against the floor echoes, followed by the relentless chiselling of tiles.

Frustration propels me out of bed. Desperate for relief from the ceaseless assault on my senses, I attempt to drown out the chaos with morning meditation and soothing music, cranking up the volume in a futile attempt to drown out the noise.

I indulge in a long shower to rouse my achy body. Escaping the clamour becomes my mission. Once dressed, I venture down the road to a quaint café, climbing a few steps to the entrance. The owner warmly greets me. I order a plate of eggs and a glass of freshly squeezed orange juice, and I remind myself to enjoy the present moment.

Afterward, I make my way to a nearby supermarket, carrying the weight of my tired body along with my beach bag as I pick up a few groceries. I contemplate heading to the beach until the wind picks up. Alas, wind is not conducive to my pain levels. Defeated, I trudge back to the apartment.

Approaching the building, I glance upward and notice a man standing on a balcony, engrossed in a loud phone conversation. "You are the culprit," I mutter, hastening my steps to seek refuge indoors and mentally prepare for the dance workshop at a hotel nearby. The hotel, a sprawling edifice, stands near a conference centre. They anticipate 600 people for the event.

The first session won't begin until the evening, so I scan the poolside for a spot to recline. The brisk wind discourages me once more.

In the bar adjacent to the lobby, I find space to indulge in some writing. My body craves sleep. If only I had a room at this hotel, I could retreat and surrender to slumber. I do my best to relax and recall the purpose for this time of rejuvenation.

I firmly believe in the healing power of dance. My ancestors, the Native Indians in Brazil, danced for various reasons: summoning rain, celebrating, initiating rituals, preparing for war, and—above all—healing. The practice of dance transcends cultures and time, connecting us all. At this conference, I will put this ancient tradition to the test, hoping it revives my weary body.

Three elegant French ladies take seats not far from me. They don't remain sitting for long. It seems they're taking full opportunity of the empty bar to practise kizomba. Observing their graceful movements distracts me from my fatigue.

I approach the ladies, estimating them to be in their forties. I introduce myself and feel warmth and kindness emanating from them. Before long, I find myself dancing with Enshabe, the lady leading the practice. My steps are clumsy, but sharing this moment invigorates me. I am happy to socialise and share a few songs, laughs, and practise my broken French.

After another unsuccessful attempt to reach the beach, thwarted by a locked gate, I end up at the 19th Hole Sports Bar for an early dinner. I sit near a small pool surrounded by palm trees as the sun gently caresses my face. Gratitude fills my heart as I savour this respite. My husband is holding down the fort at home, giving me this opportunity to be enveloped by the beauty of nature. The delicately presented salmon and broccolini with freshly squeezed orange juice is divine.

The rain holds off, and the temperature remains a comfortable 18 degrees Celsius. It's a stark contrast to the freezing weather and snow back home. Vitamin D is a precious gift, one I desperately need.

I plan to participate in two workshops: one for kizomba and another for bachata. That is my goal, but I hope to get some rest before the evening's activities begin.

"What do you need and want, Michele?" I quietly ask myself.

Sleep, my inner voice whispers in reply.

Yes, I can recharge my batteries with a little sleep before the evening event starts.

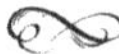

"Feel the music coursing through you," Ben, the workshop teacher and a friend of mine, says in a gentle voice. "Release your expectations; surrender to the rhythm. Dance is a sacred realm where your soul meets the melody, where your body becomes the vessel of expression." His words are a reminder to let go and embrace the unknown.

Let go ... it's a journey I'm embarking upon

Under his guidance, I step onto the crowded dance floor. Each step is a reminder to relax my shoulders and let the music cradle me. The air is alive with anticipation as we move, a sea of souls attuned to the same rhythm, each seeking their own liberation.

I wear a silk black and blue dress that mirrors the ebb and flow of kizomba. It's my pledge to immerse myself in the music, to dance for the pure joy of it. I suppress the voice that whispers doubts about my novice skills, reminding myself that everyone starts somewhere.

I gaze about the dance floor and spot a line forming. It's a line destined for Ben, the conductor of this symphony. Ana, his partner in dance and life, greets me warmly as I navigate through the throng, my heart pounding with anticipation.

Ben and another dancer engage in their steps, eyes closed, lost in the music. It's a communion of souls, a union between him, the music, and his partner. They dance as if they are the embodiment of the very notes that swirl around them.

Finally, I'm next in line. "Venha," Ben beckons me in the melodious tongue of Portugal. In his presence, I feel a camaraderie as if we've known each other for lifetimes. He understands my physical limitations and the reason I am here—to find solace and healing through dance.

"Dance is medicine," he once told me, "a remedy for the soul. Once your heart is light, your body will follow." Indeed, his words are a compass guiding me toward the uncharted shore of healing.

The music envelops us, its rhythm a heartbeat that resonates within. I stand before him, our hands entwined, our bodies poised. Our eyes lock, and the world around us fades, leaving only the music.

The kizomba beat begins its slow, deliberate cadence. We stand as one, our lower bodies performing the soft, rhythmic march in gentle unison. His hand rests firmly on the small of my back, a silent reassurance that he leads, and all I need to do is trust.

As the song progresses, I feel his guidance in every step. A step forward, a step back, a gentle sway, a shared pause—the dance is an intimate dialogue, a conversation of motion. His feet lead me here, his arm guides me there, a subtle exchange of signals. We twirl and spin, our bodies carried by the currents of music.

For a moment, doubt intrudes, a whisper of uncertainty. *What comes next?* The controlling part of me always wants to know what happens next. I stumble, then laugh.

"Relax," Ben's voice, like a gentle breeze, brushes away my worries. "Listen to the music, surrender to its current. Let the dance transport you as I guide you." His words become my anchor, and I dive back into the rhythm.

My eyes close, and suddenly, I'm adrift in a sea of sound. Every note, every beat, every inflection of the lyrics reverberates through me. The music becomes a partner in the dance, a collaborator in the choreography of my being. My body is a vessel carried by the currents of sound.

Joy surges through me. It's not merely about dancing with a skilled instructor—it's about dancing with the music itself, with the very essence of life.

The song draws to a close, merging seamlessly into another. I continue to dance with Ben, each moment a celebration of connection, of being present in the melody. This is kizomba, an intricate dialogue between souls. It's a journey of letting go, of flowing with the current, of embracing the healing power of movement.

As the night deepens and the music shifts, I'm engulfed in an urban mix of kizomba. It's different, yet familiar—a reminder that music, in all its forms, carries the promise of healing. With each step, each sway, I'm reminded of the sacrifices I've made to embrace dance therapy, to open myself to the healing energy of movement. The dance continues, and so does my journey—a dance of healing, of growth, of surrender.

My heart opens a little wider with each step, my body echoing the rhythm of life. This is my dance—a journey of release, of transformation, of community, and of becoming one with the music, the movement, and myself.

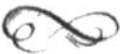

I stay in touch with four incredible French ladies from the Algarve workshops. One night, I have an online heart-to-heart with one of the ladies I hadn't connected with as much. She shares pictures of her charming city and the chateau that graces its landscape

Our conversation shifts to my health, and her kindness shines through as we discuss my book and health journey.

"I would have never suspected the battles you face," she tells me. "You don't wear it on your sleeve."

Her perception of me as radiant, happy, and joyful touches me deeply. The first night we all met in the Algarve, I observed the festivities from a distance, unable to join in because I had already pushed myself too far. In the solitude of the bathtub later that evening, tears streamed down my face as I grappled with the excruciating pain coursing through my lower back and legs.

No one knew how much time that night I spent searching for a comfortable position, struggling to find sleep amidst the turmoil. No one witnessed my brief retreats from the workshops, seeking a quiet spot to elevate my legs and close my eyes, absorbing meditations that gave me energy to keep going.

My instinct is to isolate myself, and I'm skilled at it. I don't want to burden anyone with my ordeal. Even during the workshop, I'd sneak off to the bathroom, stretch, and give my legs a rub-down to release pain and tension while offering whispered affirmations to keep smiling, to stay connected to the music's magic.

The folks I interacted with likely didn't notice my bathroom escapes. All they saw was me excusing myself and returning with a smile on my face. These hidden actions, these unspoken rituals, have simply been part of the complex journey of navigating my invisible condition in a world unaware of this invisible battle I face.

Conversing with my new French friend, I still don't reveal the whole story. How much of these intensely personal struggles should I share? The answer escapes me. I'm grateful for my innate positivity, the ability to show the bright side because that's what's beautiful to witness and experience.

Yet am I being truthful to myself?

I need to unpack this.

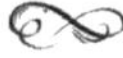

In my next therapy session, I open up about my recent solo adventure in Portugal, sharing the disconnection I feel when revealing my invisible illness to others. I tell Anne about my fear that people might not handle the situation well or know how to respond, so I often choose not to burden them.

A recurring theme surfaces—I'm afraid others won't want to be around me when I'm in pain, fearing I'll become a burden or bore them. Past comments linger: "You look perfectly fine. Are you sure it's not all in your mind?" The frequency of these kinds of comments makes me question the validity of my struggles.

But when I pause and listen to my body, it reminds me that the pain is undeniably real. It screams its existence, and I can't ignore it.

Anne interjects with valuable insight. "By withholding the truth from acquaintances and new friends, you deny them the opportunity to make their own choices. You're trying to anticipate their reactions, but that's beyond your control. Each person must navigate their own path, and how they handle your news is entirely up to them. You don't have to shoulder that burden; it's theirs to bear."

Her words resonate. In my attempts to present my best self, I'm not exactly being true to who I am. Acknowledging that people dislike chronic complainers, I admit to Anne that I avoid sharing my struggles—even with my children—not wanting them to carry that burden or have a negative impression of me.

Anne stresses the idea that by not disclosing my true state, I might be hindering the ability of others to be vulnerable with me. I'm signalling that my struggles are off-limits, preventing others from offering their support. By sharing my struggles, I am showing that I trust them with this knowledge, expressing my desire for them to know how important they are to me.

"Don't you think there should be a balance?" I ask.

"What does that look like for you?" Anne presses.

I consider her question for a minute before answering. "I think it involves openness, a willingness to let people see the real me, even when it's not all sunshine. I trust that this illness has a purpose, a lesson, a reason. I hope it won't define my entire existence."

My thoughts come together as I voice them aloud. "It's an opportunity to appreciate life, cherish its moments, and unearth the essence of who I am. There's a real 'me,' a version of myself that's been relegated to the background, in need of tender loving care, compassion, grace, and vulnerability. It's a slow process, a delicate connection I'm striving to make, but I believe I'll get there."

Anne nods in agreement. "Balance comes when you can listen to your needs and give that a voice, too."

I appreciate the reminder that to be heard, I must first listen to my own needs and stay truthful to myself.

By the end of the session, I feel more at ease with this inner tension of how much of my health struggles to reveal, and to whom. It is yet another thing that I cannot fully answer, but I am growing comfortable with the uncertainty.

Once again, I feel grateful for how music is becoming such an instrument in lifting my spirit, giving me hope and, most of all, serving as an avenue to finding community and shared passion. It's a way to push myself out of the isolation

I have been falling into. I am truly grateful for the combination of my therapy sessions, dance therapy, and friendships—together, they are providing a healing balm to my soul.

Maybe it's a midlife crisis brought about by turning 40, but I just want to connect with others who love music and dance because it really lifts me up! I have great plans for my upcoming journey to France, envisioning a chance to deepen connections and explore the connections that dance and shared experiences create for healing.

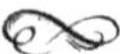

I'm thrilled to be on this exhilarating adventure in Angers, France. Friends I made at the dance conference in Algarve invited me to join them for a dance workshop featuring an astounding couple from Lyon.

The journey commences on a Thursday afternoon when Marie Ange, one of my newfound friends, picks me up from Nantes, over an hour away. Her caring gesture instantly warms my heart, especially since we only interacted for a few days during the previous conference. Now here I am, staying at her place, feeling excited and grateful for her hospitality.

Despite my unpredictable health conditions, I set expectations high for myself when travelling or meeting new people. Marie Ange's warmth and motherly nature put me at ease. She's considerate and thoughtful, even asking about my food preferences.

The French people's love for bread and cheese are a delightful change from the norm. Even though the timing of meals is different, I soak in every moment. The first evening, I spend time with Marie Ange's family—her partner and two daughters. We chat late into the night, and I retire to her oldest daughter's room for rest. The room is decorated with memories of the girl's travels, invoking a sense of wanderlust.

However, my body decides to act up, reminding me of my health challenges as I struggle to find a comfortable position to sleep. Eventually, through prayer and meditation, I manage to find some reprieve.

Friday morning arrives, and I wake up to the sound of life bustling in the house. My body feels tense, and my pelvic area is cramping, adding to the pain I constantly face. Despite this, I gather the courage to reveal the truth of my current pain level to Marie Ange, and she responds with kindness and understanding.

We venture into Angers' town centre on a sunny morning with clear blue skies. Marie Ange is planning her wedding, which is taking place in a few months, and I am invited to join her at a bridal shop. I'm touched to accompany my new friend as she tries on wedding dresses. After some sightseeing, we enjoy ice cream by a fountain.

Later in the evening, we have dinner with the core volunteers and the stars of the dance workshop. I feel welcomed by this dancing community despite my outsider status. The camaraderie, laughter, and jokes create an atmosphere of joy I relish being a part of, even if it's mostly in French and I can't understand it all.

As the night winds down, I lie in bed, allowing myself to feel the pain my body is experiencing. I remind myself of the love and affection I received throughout the day, drinking in these acts of kindness as medicine for my soul.

The next morning, I wake up feeling a bit better and join Marie Ange for breakfast. She's already prepared pizza and carrot cake to share with other volunteers. We head to the venue to set up for the event, where we'll come together once more as a dancing community.

In the evening, a band from the Dominican Republic performs live, and the dance floor comes alive with couples dancing, smiling, and singing along. The atmosphere is contagious, and the rhythm is infectious. I watch and soak it all in. Every now and then, I am asked to dance, and it feels magical. Merengue, salsa, bachata, and, of course, kizomba, fill the air. I am touched to be here, grateful for the sense of belonging and camaraderie I feel.

Despite my disabilities and health challenges, the love and care I receive and the moments of joy and laughter make this journey unforgettable.

Chapter 27

Aftermath, A Formidable Beast

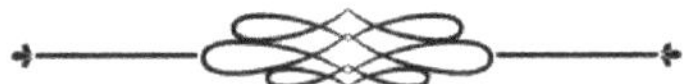

"Are you ready for this?" my friend asks, her expression a mix of concern and excitement.

I offer her a weak smile, questioning the wisdom of my decision. "I'm as ready as I'll ever be." We walk into Thomond Park Stadium for an Ed Sheeran concert.

I try to pace myself, securing a seat in the arena, acknowledging my dwindling stamina, but that is just one piece of the puzzle. The colossal sea of people and their cacophony, the deafening music from speakers pounding with bass—an overwhelming cascade of sensations engulf me as I make my way to my seat.

In my earlier days, such overwhelming stimuli never posed a problem. I relished concerts growing up, but my illness had sentenced me to a concertless existence. Until now. Ed Sheeran's music strikes a chord in my heart, and the fact that he is holding a concert here in Limerick is a dream come true.

A concert in Dublin is too far for my aching body, but this—this I couldn't resist. I acquired the tickets a year in advance, a present to myself, a promise that I would still savour life's pleasures. I brought ear plugs, an attempt to temper the auditory assault, yet didn't anticipate the many other challenges waiting for me.

I arrive at the venue with a throbbing tension headache behind my eyes, especially on the left side, but refuse to let it become a leash around my joy. A chicken panini and a glass of wine for dinner helped, but only slightly. I won't falter now, not after I finally made it here.

I immerse myself in the show, singing along, employing deep breaths to cope with the pain, occasionally covering my face with both hands, gently massaging pressure points, even sneaking in a bit of EFT Tapping during the songs—anything to distract from the escalating pain coursing through my body.

My friend leans closer. "Are you okay?"

"I'm managing," I reply, my voice faltering slightly. "It's just... intense."

My friend offers a supportive smile before turning her attention back to the stage. As the concert progresses, Ed Sheeran's music becomes a lifeline in the tumult of sensations. The rhythmic beats are an anchor guiding me through the storm. The crowd's energy, a force of its own, resonates with me. I find comfort in specific songs, like "Photograph" and "Thinking Out Loud," each note a balm to my aching soul.

The emotional highs are palpable, another reminder of the healing power of music. The lows, however, are equally intense, as my body wages a silent war against the physical strain. My friend asks me again if I want to leave. My resounding NO is unwavering. I am staying... I can endure this.

And endure I do.

Mixed emotions swirl within me as the concert concludes. Delight and the thrill of sharing this experience with my friend intertwine with the battle I wage against the pain, now a formidable beast. I hold onto her arm tightly as we navigate through the throngs of people, the stadium's 30,000 souls descending upon Limerick's streets.

"You okay?" she asks again, glancing at me.

I manage a nod, my lips trembling as I force a smile. "Yeah, just need to get through the crowd."

My disappointment is acute when we reach the bus stop only to learn the bus is going to be a 1.2 km trek away. A small distance to some, but with my dwindling energy, it feels like an arduous journey. We trudge on, my back and neck crying out and my migraine now a blazing inferno.

"Can you make it?" my friend asks as she holds my arms.

"We have to," I reply, pushing myself forward. "Just a little longer. There is no way anyone can drive through this crowd."

At last, we reach the buses, and I find a spot on the front seat. The driver's frustration at being relocated by the authorities from the original stop only adds to the disarray. The bus finally starts moving at 11:45 pm, the city congested with folks returning to their vehicles or converging on the local pubs.

I make it home past midnight, a shower my first respite. I try to persuade myself into sleep, but comfort remains elusive. I toss and turn, drifting into brief spells of slumber, only to be jolted awake.

This same night, Ryan is volunteering with the Order of Malta for a Darkness into Light event, and Anthony is driving him. They need to be there at 3:15 am. I hear my husband rise and—hours later—return home, these small disturbances gnawing at my rest.

I remain in bed through the morning and beyond, but my obligations loom large. "Feeling any better?" Anthony's voice reaches me as he enters the room. I already cancelled flower shopping with him three times.

I muster a weak smile, my eyes heavy. "Not really. But I'm trying."

He nods. "Take your time."

The day is bathed in glorious sunlight, a stark contrast to how I feel inside. I still haven't recovered from the concert, but I push myself to get ready and head out shopping with my husband.

"You sure you're up for this?" Anthony asks. I note the familiar concern in his voice.

"I promise," I reply with determination. "I'm not going to back out this time."

Sunglasses shielding my light-sensitive eyes, I navigate the shopping as swiftly as I can. Decision-making feels like a marathon, my agony a constant reminder that I can't just push through like I could in the past. I finally admit defeat and retreat home, leaving our newly acquired flowers outside. At least they'll enjoy the nourishing rain.

I curl up in a foetal position, listening to various meditations, practicing breathing techniques, desperately trying to rest. Saturday night offers no relief as pain's grasp tightens further. By 5 am, I can't endure the pain any longer. I vomit whatever is in my stomach. I barely have the strength to turn on the shower, but the cascading water provides a momentary distraction from the pounding headache, persistent nausea, and burning sensations coursing through my back, legs, and face.

"Are you okay in there?" Anthony's voice echoes through the bathroom door.

"Just … dealing with the aftermath," I manage to respond.

He doesn't say anything further, but I know he understands the unspoken struggle I face. I try to be as gentle with myself as my husband is with me—acknowledging the triumph of attending the concert in my pursuit of normalcy while also acknowledging that rest is essential.

Sunday dawns, but my world remains cloaked in shadows, my eyes acutely sensitive to light. I lie in bed, guilt gnawing at me for not being present with my boys.

"Mom, you should come outside," Ryan calls from outside the bedroom, enthusiasm in his voice.

"I wish I could, sweetheart," I reply. "But I need to recover."

Anthony offers to take me to the pool, a place where my body usually finds surcease. This time, however, boisterous youngsters in the water drive me out after only a few minutes. At least I ventured out of the house.

On Monday, it's nearly 1 pm by the time I manage to emerge from bed and dress for the day. The relentless grip of my headache, though not the "lightning zaps" I felt over the last couple of days, still clings to my forehead and eyes. Nausea sweeps over me in waves.

Was it worth it? Worth days of agonizing recovery for a concert of just a few hours?

A paradoxical answer emerges, a blend of yes and no.

Yes, it was splendid reliving a past joy of attending concerts to rekindle the embers of my old self. The rhythmic beats became a beacon guiding me through the storm of pain, and specific songs were a balm to my aching soul.

And no, my body's resilience was lower than I'd expected; it took far longer to reach equilibrium than I'd anticipated. It sapped more from me than I'd realised. The aftermath was a formidable beast.

This serves as yet another lesson in my ongoing journey, a perpetual navigation of living with an invisible illness. The well of energy within me often appears deeper than it truly is. My desire to give, to embrace life's experiences, is boundless. Reality is another thing all together.

"I don't think I'll be going to another show anytime soon," I say to my friend over the phone, "unless I have the luxury of a couple of weeks of rest afterward, and even then, I might not brave the entirety of the show as I did this time."

"It's all about finding that balance, isn't it?" she agrees.

Chapter 28

Closing in on the Cause

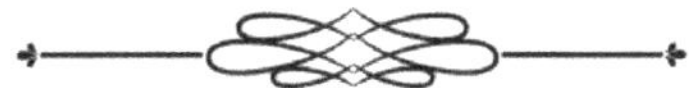

More than two years have elapsed since the pandemic began, and nearly four years since the onset of my invisible illness. Dr. Ryan, my consultant neurologist who once offered a glimmer of hope, is no longer working at the hospital. His absence leaves a void.

Now in September 2022, my husband stands by my side as we finally return to University Hospital Limerick, the setting of my prior hopes and frustrations. As I approach the reception desk at the outpatient department, I am told Dr. Kelly is the new consultant neurologist.

Before long, Dr. Kelly greets us and leads the way into his office. "Please, have a seat. Let's talk about how you've been feeling." The room is a simple yet functional space—a large desk at the centre holding a few files, an examination bed with a paper cover on my right side and filing cabinets with books to my left. Above the examination bed, bottles of disinfectant stand alongside machines and other medical equipment.

Despite its clinical air, the room emanates calm. Dr. Kelly's voice is warm, with a strong accent that somehow helps to ease my tension—a tension that has built up over two years of waiting to be reviewed.

My husband, always a steady presence, adds, "We've been navigating through these challenges for quite a while now. Any insight you can provide will be immensely helpful."

Dr. Kelly listens intently as I give him a rundown of the last few years with this condition. He nods, seeming to understand the complexities of my journey. "I want to get to the bottom of this," he assures. I sense his sincerity and am encouraged at a promise of renewed attention to my case. He suggests new MRI brain scans with contrast and a brain MRA as well, an effort to unravel the mysteries lurking beneath the surface.

"Let's schedule these scans urgently. The new machines we now have are top-of-the-line, providing a more detailed look," Dr. Kelly explains as he types out a request for the scans on his computer. He knows I have facial pain and that my condition has been labelled as trigeminal neuralgia. "A new brain scan might show the root cause of the pain and from there, a course of treatment."

I am grateful for his commitment to finding the root cause and walk out of the consultation feeling lighter, glad that things are moving in the right direction. He promised to see me again, at the latest, in two months.

I try calling the MRI department yet again to secure an appointment for a scan. The pandemic has created a backlog, and the appointment date remains elusive after two months of phone calls.

"It's like waiting for the clouds to part and reveal the sun," I tell my husband, trying to convey the mix of anticipation and frustration that colours this wait.

Persistence becomes my ally as I navigate the bureaucratic maze. I try to be patient. This journey has been so long, I can wait a bit longer. I cannot see my neurologist without the results of the scan, and without these, I am not sure what course to take next!

When March 2023 rolls around, I am informed that my referral has been lost. Part of me snaps. The secretary, understanding my predicament, manages to secure an appointment for May. Two more months of waiting. Patience is not just a virtue but a necessity in this journey towards finding answers.

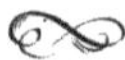

The day of the long-awaited brain MRI finally arrives. As I step into the sterile room, a chill raises goosebumps on my skin. The technician, clad in scrubs and a mask, guides me through the process.

The coldness of the room feels like it's seeping into my bones as I lie down on the examination bed. A head strap secures my head and neck into an unnatural posture. The room echoes with the hum of machinery, and the stark white walls seem to close in.

"Are you okay?" the technician asks as he checks my earmuffs and strap.

"Yes, thank you," I respond. "Please, take your time. I've waited so long for this MRI. Make sure to capture as many images as needed." This MRI is my best chance for answers. I'm here for a revelation, not a mere scan.

Entering the narrow tube, I feel claustrophobia creeping in. The space is tight, and the machine's relentless drumming intensifies my anxiety. I focus on my breathing, attempting to regulate my heartbeat. The cool air in the room collides with the warmth of my breath, a silent struggle within the confined space. The technician's voice, barely audible through the headphones, offers periodic reassurances that become a lifeline in the disorienting void.

As the rhythmic clunks and buzzes of the MRI machine begin, I find comfort in my chosen distraction—classical music. The soothing melodies offer a temporary escape from the confinement of the machine.

Emerging from the tube, the chill hits me once again. The technician prepares me for the next phase—a needle piercing my left arm, injecting contrast dye into my veins. A metallic taste floods my mouth as the dye courses through my bloodstream.

Back in the tube, the second round begins. The machine resumes its symphony, capturing images with relentless precision. I clutch the emergency button, a lifeline that I dare not press. The seconds stretch into minutes, the minutes into what feels like an hour, maybe longer. This confinement becomes a test of resilience. With each passing moment, I battle the rising fear, the urge to press that button and escape the metallic jaws of the machine.

Finally, after an intense one hour and 20 minutes, the machine falls silent. The ordeal is over. I'm left with a mix of exhaustion and relief. But surely the comprehensive scans have left no stone unturned. I leave the hospital with a quiet optimism, a glimmer of hope that these images will unlock the answers I've been seeking for so long.

Three days after the MRI, I'm sitting outside on my porch. The sun is bright, the air calm. I'm in the middle of meditating, focusing on the rhythm of my breath, when my phone rings.

"Hello?" I answer quickly, still half in the peaceful world I'd created for myself.

On the other end, I hear the familiar voice of my neurologist. "Hi, Michele, this is Dr. Kelly. I've got your MRI results. How are you feeling?"

"Hi, Doctor. Thanks for calling. I'm feeling ... okay, I suppose." A hint of apprehension creeps in. Why is he calling me? Is there bad news?

"Well," he continues, "I wanted to talk to you before you get a letter from the neurosurgeon, so you're not caught off guard."

"Okay ..." I reply, the tension building up quickly.

"So, your problem is mechanical," he says, with a slight chuckle, as if relieved to have figured something out.

"Mechanical? What does that mean?" I stand, clutching my phone tightly.

"The MRI showed very clearly what's causing the pain in your trigeminal nerve," he explains, his voice almost too cheerful. "It's mechanical, which means something can be done about it. No wonder the medication didn't work for you!"

I start pacing, trying to wrap my mind around what he's saying. Of course the medication didn't work for me, I think to myself.

The doctor's voice pulls me back. "Would you like me to refer you to a private neurosurgeon or a public one?"

"What do you mean? Why do I need a neurosurgeon?" My heart races as the reality of the situation begins to set in.

"Well, it's mechanical," he repeats, as if that explains everything. "They can perform an operation, and you'll feel better again. You won't have your trigeminal nerve pain anymore."

"Oh ..." It feels like the ground is shifting beneath me. I look around the porch, trying to anchor myself in the familiar surroundings. "How long will it take to see someone in the public sector?" I ask, desperate for some sense of control.

"I'm not sure. The waiting list could vary, but this would be for an operation, like--"

"What operation?" I interrupt, my anxiety mounting.

"An MVD," he says matter-of-factly. "Yes, most likely a microvascular decompression. The MRI shows a very clear picture of it."

"All right ..." I try to stay calm. "And do you know how long it would take with a private hospital?"

"No, I'm not sure about that either."

"Okay ... can you send the referral to the public hospital first? Let's see what they have to say."

"Sure," he replies. "I'll do that, so you don't have to see me again. Now you're in the hands of the neurosurgeon."

After the call ends, I stand still on the porch, trying to centre myself by focusing on the feeling of the sun on my skin, but my mind is racing. What just happened? My neurologist had talked so fast, so excitedly. Mechanical ... great. It took four and a half years to find out there's something pressing on my nerve.

And I need surgery? What the hell?

I force myself to breathe, to ground myself. I walk over to the grass, slip off my shoes, and let my feet sink into the earth. I take a few deep breaths, trying to steady the whirlwind in my mind. I'm happy but terrified.

What does this all mean? Why couldn't the doctor ask me to come in, to talk to me in person instead of over the phone? I could barely understand him with his accent and how fast he was speaking.

Okay, fine. Maybe I'm being pedantic ... I am grateful. But how long will this take?

A few weeks later, I call the neurologist's office, asking for the phone number of the hospital they referred me to in Cork. After some time, I finally get through. The news isn't what I hoped for—I'm on an "urgent" waiting list to see the neurosurgeon, and it's a three-year wait.

Three years.

Frustrated, I hang up and immediately call the neurologist's secretary again. "Could you please ask the doctor to make a referral for the private hospital? I want to see Dr. O'Brien." I ask for a doctor who is supposed to be the top expert in trigeminal neuralgia in Ireland. I heard about him through the Facial Pain Association in the States and a Facebook group I follow.

The secretary is kind and agrees. I don't have to wait long—just three months before I finally get to see the private neurosurgeon. It's a lot better than three years.

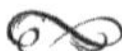

My husband and I step through the doors of the private Hermitage Clinic; it's a bit like walking into an elegant hotel. Plush couches grace the foyer, and a vibrant coffee shop on the upper floor beckons with lively colours, a stark contrast to the hushed atmosphere. Approaching the reception desk, I inquire about the neurosurgeon's office.

"Take the elevator to the basement level and head left to door three," the receptionist instructs politely. As we move toward the elevator, a peculiar slowness in my thoughts sets in, perhaps due to the fatigue from the two-hour journey or the weight of the unknown.

Intentionally leaving the pink folder containing my documents, tests, and reports in the car, I carry only the MRI CD—a small disc holding the key to unravelling my pain. The elevator doors part, and we turn left as instructed. The plush carpet underfoot muffles our footsteps, oddly comforting. A constellation of consultation rooms sprawls ahead, each like a door to a unique universe of possibilities.

A gentle nudge from my husband behind me provides the comfort I need to proceed.

In the waiting area, two ladies sit to my left, and a couple in front of me are deep in conversation. To the right, a glass window frames two secretaries. A countertop notice catches my eye: "Dr. McCarthy's secretary" pointing left and "Mr. O'Brien's secretary" pointing right.

I hesitate. The secretary raises her window, bringing my attention back to the present.

"Name." Her voice carries a tinge of impatience.

"Michele Roys."

"And who are you here to see?"

"Dr. O'Brien," I respond.

The secretary directs me to a seat before lowering the window. Choosing a wooden chair in the corner, starkly contrasting the opulent lobby seating, I settle in. My thoughts churn.

"You might want to jot down your questions now." My husband's gaze remains fixed on his phone, scrolling through notifications and reminders. I nod, grateful for his presence and practicality. Retrieving a notepad from my purse, I write a few questions I have for the doctor.

What's your opinion? Can you interpret my MRI? Am I a candidate for MVD operation? What are the risks?

Time drifts by. The two ladies on my left are summoned. I'm next in line. The waiting room sees more arrivals. One of the newcomers sits near me.

"I am sorry to interrupt," she says, "but who are you here to see?"

"Dr. O'Brien," I answer.

She smiles warmly. "You're in good hands; he's a remarkable doctor. I owe my recovery to him." Her enthusiasm is contagious, filing me with reassurance.

"Do you have TN?" I ask. She shakes her head and tells me about her aneurysm, an ensuing operation, and the tumultuous backdrop of Covid. Another lady joins the conversation and tells of her struggle with TN. An instant connection surges between us; even her face mirrors my own battles—no makeup, cautious movements to appease the pain's demands.

I am not alone. Our conversations are immediately deep, and we are candid about the depths of pain, the limits of medications, and the haunting spectre of suicidal thoughts.

"How long have you had TN?" I ask.

"I'm going on 18 months of hell with it," she reveals, a voice edged with weariness.

"You will find a way," I assure her.

"How long have you had it?" she then asks.

"Nearly five years now." Memories of these past years, the various avenues of treatment, the struggle for answers, and the slow journey toward acceptance all swirl within me. "I am now managing it without medications, more of a holistic approach." My words carry a glimmer of triumph.

The door's swing announces my turn, and I bid farewell to my newfound companions. Stepping into the doctor's office, I carry their stories with me, a tapestry of pain and hope that has woven our lives together in a few brief moments of discussing our common journeys.

Dr. O'Brien extends a welcoming hand, ushering my husband and me into his office. A computer sits on his desk, and a bookshelf stands behind it. A window in the corner offers a view of the manicured lawn outside. My husband takes a seat beside me. His presence grounds me.

"So, you're here for facial pain." He holds a pen, ready to capture the contours of my narrative. I relate my journey—the onset of pain, the relentless passage of four years and nine months marked by countless visits to doctors and neurologists.

He continues asking me questions and I answer, sharing about my pain triggers—how the wind's touch can unleash agony, how a scarf has become a barrier against the pain.

I hand him the CD.

Dr. O'Brien's fingers dance over the keyboard, the computer's screen flickering to life as he inserts the MRI CD. The labyrinth of my anatomy unfolds before me, and I see the intricate pathways of pain visualised for the first time. I don't understand what I'm seeing at first.

Dr. O'Brien's focus hones on a specific image. "This is your trigeminal nerve, and here," he points, "the superior cerebellar artery loops around it, touching both sides."

I blink as a moment of sudden clarity descends. It is as though the puzzle pieces of the last five years are suddenly falling into place. There it is, the source of my torment, unveiled.

"This is what's causing your pain. Are you open to fixing it?"

I look at my husband. He takes my hand, squeezing it reassuringly. I know the look on his face. This is my journey, and the decision before me is mine as well.

"Yes," I say hesitantly, "but what kind of procedure would this be?"

He explains what it would entail—something called a microvascular decompression (MVD) procedure. The steps are intricate, as any such surgical procedure would be.

"Risks are inherent in any procedure," Dr. O'Brien adds, "facial paralysis, hearing loss, nerve damage, unmanageable bleeding under anaesthesia. Your decision should be informed. Our TN patients yearn for relief. We cannot promise pain-free days, but we strive for the best possible outcome."

I stand at a crossroads, fear and hope entwined.

"You deserve a life without pain," he states. "The choice is yours. Continue your holistic approach or venture toward a more lasting solution."

The promise of surgery holds an allure, for sure. The possibility of total healing? Yet doubts also cast shadows as faces flash in my mind—my two boys, mostly—and I think of the worst that could happen to me.

"Will my condition worsen without surgery?" I ask.

He answers with analogy. "Think of a dripping tap, how over time, it can erode stone. This is similar to your nerve's gradual erosion over time if you leave things as they are."

The consultation draws to a close, and Dr. O'Brien lets us know he'll send a comprehensive cost breakdown. I know that our next steps will also depend on those numbers.

Leaving through the waiting room, I see the two ladies still sitting side by side.

"Best of luck to both of you," I say.

I step out of the hospital, and a whirlwind of emotions envelopes me as real as the wind outside. Did I ask the right questions? Did I miss something? My husband takes my hand once more.

"We'll figure this out," he said. "You've come so far, and I can't say how much I admire you for this battle you've fought."

His steadying presence offers comfort. Yes, we'll move forward, together.

At home that evening, thoughts swirl within me. The flicker of hope coexists with a gnawing uncertainty. I don't want to have to undergo a delicate surgery that potentially has dire consequences. I wish I could be an exception to the rule.

Yet I feel relief at the validation that has eluded me for years. I have confirmation that my pain is not a phantom. The image on the screen—a nerve ensnared by an artery—stands as irrefutable proof.

My pain has a tangible root, and my struggle is real. Yet, it doesn't explain the pain in the rest of my body. The weight of a decision hangs heavily on my mind.

It is a high-wire act between potential relief and the dangers that surgery presents. All the dire possibilities the doctor outlined echo in my mind.

With each inhale and exhale, I seek comfort, a rhythm to steady this inner storm. My breath becomes a lifeline, guiding me through the turmoil.

Yet, amid the chaos, a whisper of reassurance emerges—a belief that the answers reside within me, waiting to unfurl like petals in due time. I trust that God, with his unfathomable wisdom, will reveal what I need to know, one step at a time.

I will wait on the surgery for now and follow my intuition that there is still more my body is trying to reveal. I need only to trust the journey, to let the pages of my story turn, and to embrace the narrative as it unfolds.

Chapter 29

Progress, Not Perfection

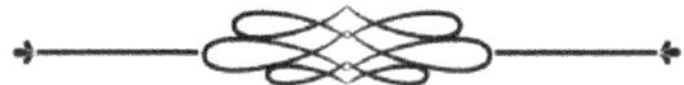

The dance of healing unfolds. I sway between vulnerability and strength, between acknowledging wounds of my past and embracing the resilience within. Each therapy session, each fumbling step on this arduous road, is a choreography of self-discovery. It's a delicate balance of facing the pain and finding comfort in moments of self-care.

As the melody of life plays on, I continue to honour my commitment, nurturing my growth and well-being. I celebrate the progress I make, no matter how small, finally understanding that healing is not a linear path. There will be setbacks and challenges, but I will persevere, armed with the resilience I've cultivated.

I give myself permission to stumble, to learn, and to forgive.

And so, with each session, each moment of self-compassion, I take another step forward on this intricate dance floor of healing. I learn to trust myself, honour my needs, and embrace the journey, however long it may take. In this dance, I find freedom to be vulnerable, to heal, and to reclaim all the parts of myself that were lost along the way.

I am a dancer in the grand ballet of life, moving through the steps of self-discovery and healing. With every graceful movement, I release the weight of the past and the burdens that have held me back. I twirl and spin, letting go of self-criticism and embracing self-love. In this dance, I find strength, resilience, and the power to shape my own narrative.

I navigate the intricate choreography of healing, knowing that with each step, I am reclaiming my true self. I honour the journey, the progress—not perfection—and the transformation unfolding before me. As I move through this beautiful dance, I am filled with hope, knowing that one day, I will fully embrace the freedom and joy that come from healing and self-discovery.

The music plays and I dance.

Epilogue

Thank you for taking the time to read my story. I hope it has inspired you in your own journey as you seek the answers that resonate with your heart. While this book covers my experiences only up to mid-2023, I'd like to share a brief update on what has been happening from then until the time of writing this epilogue—late 2024.

My quest for answers continued, and a nagging feeling that something was missing in my health puzzle proved to be right. In early 2024, my blood tests were sent to a specialized lab in Germany, and I was diagnosed with Lyme disease.

While I still don't know where or when I contracted it, that's not my main focus right now. What matters most is nourishing my body and continuing the healing process. The tools I've gathered along my journey are the same ones I'm applying as I navigate this new chapter.

Maybe I'll write about this next stage of my journey someday—the treatments, the diagnosis, and the ongoing challenge of being the CEO of my own body. It's about truly listening to what my body needs so I can align with my true self once again.

I'm grateful that my determination has led me to answers and paths I might have missed if I had given up or simply accepted what was first told to me. Right now, I've decided to hold off on surgery for the trigeminal neuralgia to give my body time to heal while I treat the Lyme disease. I trust this will help with the inflammation and perhaps ease the intensity of my symptoms. I have faith that God will provide a way forward and give me strength to keep going, even through the fatigue, aches, and facial pain.

My new mission is unfolding—a deep and heartfelt desire to empower women who face chronic pain and invisible illness, helping them rediscover their joy and inner strength so they can lead vibrant, fulfilling lives despite the obstacles in their way.

Remember: You have that strength within you, too. Keep pushing forward, find your joy, and allow yourself to live life to the fullest—that's our true calling!

ACKNOWLEDGEMENTS

In the journey of chronic illness, no one walks alone. This book exists because of countless hearts that held space for my pain, hands that lifted me up, and voices that reminded me to keep going when the darkness felt overwhelming.

To my husband Anthony, who has been my rock for twenty odd years—your unwavering love and support have been my greatest medicine. To my boys, Collin and Ryan, who've grown into young men watching their mother battle invisible enemies—your understanding, help, and the joy you bring to my life have been more healing than any prescription.

To Bethany Kelly, my developmental coach from Publishing Partners who was not just my first reader but my first cheerleader—your candid feedback and constant encouragement helped shape both these pages and my confidence as a writer. Your faithful reminders to keep going inspired me to share my message.

To my editor Bonita Jewel, thank you for your patience and encouragement, as well as your meticulous attention to detail that caught things I would have missed and made this long process easier for me. Thank you for being part of my story and helping me bring this book to life.

To my incredible beta readers—Craig McKeown, Dr. Eimear Kelly, my brother Andre Felipe, and sister Clara Galvao—who dedicated their time and energy to reading my drafts. Your thoughtful feedback transformed this book. Each of you brought unique perspectives that enriched this narrative: Craig, for your honest feedback to help me see how other readers might view it and ensure it made sense for them; Dr. Eimear, for giving that insight from a doctor's perspective and ensuring the details were accessible yet authentic; Andre, for helping me find the balance between hope and raw honesty; and Clara, for your emotional insights that helped me dig deeper into the harder parts of this story. Your marginal notes, lengthy emails, and passionate discussions about this story showed me what was possible.

To the remarkable individuals who graciously endorsed this book—Kris Carr, Dr. Petra Frese, Macarena luz Bianchi, Mina Grace Ward, Carol Register, Kristin Ericksen and Lia Valencia Key—your words of support mean more than you know. Your willingness to stand behind this story helps ensure it reaches those who need it most. Thank you for using your platforms and influence to amplify the voices of chronic illness warriors.

To my family—my grandmother, Benedita Teles, for your devotion, perseverance, and grace while you face so many ailments with such resilience. You have taught me to keep going and trust that God would bring the best through these tests. To my mother Tania, for your fortitude and love. Thank you for teaching me to appreciate flowers, art, dance, and music, and find joy in the little things. To my siblings, Clara, Mariane, Andre, Anderson, and Angelo, I love you so much and I am so grateful for your support and belief in me through the years. To my uncles Francisco and Carlos Alberto, whose strength, wisdom, and example have inspired me throughout my life—thank you for showing me what resilience looks like.

To my faith community, especially Eloise, Jeanette, David, Chengetai and Anthony, Tobi, Mable, Dawn, Lloyd, Karina, Laura, Bryan and Ruth, Sean and Mary, and John and Sarah—your prayers have carried me through countless dark nights. The grace of God has been my anchor, manifested through your continuous support and love.

To my dear friends who have walked this journey with me: Ana Flavia and Rodrigo, Nishant, Tania, Emer, Terence and Sophia, Craig, Aisling and Andrew, for your years of faithful friendship and check-ins. Rita, for seeing me through so many seasons and ensuring I always look fab. Mary Dunphy and Denis Creighton, for your friendship, insights, and unwavering belief in me. Tom Bryant, for helping solidify the title of the book and showing such faith and trust in my vision. Marie Ange and Stefan, Raji, Theresa, Mary, Mindy, Elisse, Haaris, Marystela, Paddy, Deb (and kiddoes), and Martin C.—you've texted, called, shown up with meals, shared laughter, hugs, and offered shoulders to cry on. You've demonstrated that true friendship doesn't require perfect health or endless energy. Your grace in accepting my limitations while celebrating my victories has taught me how to be a better friend to myself.

To those who believed in me when I was growing up and inspired me to keep going and supported me in my many adventures— tio Vilmar and tia Lucia, Samuel, Julian, John, Kalli, Jon Karlson, David and Hema, Nilsa, Marli, Jair and Marcia—thank you for seeing something I couldn't see in myself and for giving me the confidence to keep following my dreams. To those who made a lasting impression and have already gone to their heavenly reward—Jon C., Angelina (a.k.a. 'mama'), and Paul H.—you inspired me to be a better person and keep smiling through my pain. Thank you!

To my therapists (you know who you are), holistic healers, and practitioners who have been instrumental in my journey.

To my fellow chronic pain warriors—those I've met in person, online communities, and through this journey—your courage inspires me daily. Every story shared, every tear witnessed, every triumph celebrated has contributed to the tapestry of hope this book aims to weave.

To the trail blazers, who shared their stories, persevered and now show that it can be done, thank you for creating your podcasts, books and courses to help us believe in ourselves: Kris Carr, Ed Mylett, Jamie Kern Lima, Kristin Neff, Jen Gottlieb, Gabby Bernstein, Brene Brown, Dr. Mark Hyman, and so many more to name.

To my dance community, thank you for keeping the music playing even on days when my steps were uncertain. The joy of Latin dancing has been my reminder that life's beauty persists despite pain.

Finally, to every reader holding this book—thank you for allowing me to share this journey with you. May you find here what you need most: whether it's understanding, hope, or the reminder that joy can coexist with pain.

With a heart filled with gratitude & gratefulness,

Michele

Resources

Trigeminal Neuralgia Support:

Trigeminal Neuralgia Association (TNA): https://www.tna.org

The TNA offers support, education, and resources for people diagnosed with Trigeminal Neuralgia and facial pain disorders.

Facial Pain Association: https://www.facialpain.org

This organization provides information, community support, and treatment options for individuals suffering from Trigeminal Neuralgia and related conditions.

Invisible Illness & Chronic Pain:

The Mighty: https://themighty.com

A platform where people with chronic illnesses, including invisible diseases and chronic pain, share stories and find support from others.

Pain Connection (US Pain Foundation): https://www.painconnection.org

Pain Connection is a program of the U.S. Pain Foundation, providing resources, peer support, and training for chronic pain sufferers and their families.

Trigeminal Neuralgia Association UK (TNA UK): https://www.tna.org.uk

TNA UK provides support, information, and advocacy for individuals affected by Trigeminal Neuralgia across the United Kingdom.

Trigeminal Neuralgia Ireland Support Group

Facebook Group: https://www.facebook.com/groups/TNIreland

A closed Facebook group specifically for people in Ireland who suffer from Trigeminal Neuralgia to share experiences and support.

UK Trigeminal Neuralgia Support Group

Facebook Group:https://www.facebook.com/groups/UKTNsupport

A Facebook support group for individuals living with TN in the UK, providing a platform for sharing advice and stories.

Lyme Disease Support:

Global Lyme Alliance: https://globallymealliance.org

A research-driven organization dedicated to conquering Lyme and other tick-borne diseases, providing support and education to those affected.

LymeDisease.org: https://www.lymedisease.org

A patient advocacy organization that provides educational resources, research, and a community for Lyme disease patients.

Books for Further Reading

- Brown, Brené. *The Gifts of Imperfection: Let Go of Who You Think You're Supposed to Be and Embrace Who You Are*. Hazelden Publishing, 2010.
    - A powerful exploration of vulnerability, courage, and self-compassion by renowned researcher Brené Brown.
- Carr, Kris. *Crazy Sexy Diet: Eat Your Veggies, Ignite Your Spark, and Live Like You Mean It!* Skirt, 2011.
- Carr, Kris. *I'm Not a Mourning Person: Braving Loss, Grief, and the Big Messy Emotions That Happen When Life Falls Apart,* Hay House 2023.
    - Kris Carr's wellness and lifestyle advice includes the Inner Circle Wellness Program, which can be accessed through her website: https://kriscarr.com
- Collison, Lily. Grit: *The Power of Passion and Perseverance for Chronic Illness.* CreateSpace Independent Publishing, 2017.
    - A guide on finding strength and resilience when faced with chronic conditions.
- Gottlieb, Jen. *Be Seen: Find Your Voice, Build Your Brand, Live Your Dream*. Hay House, 2023.
    - Jen Gottlieb shares her personal journey of transformation and offers actionable advice for achieving visibility and impact.

- Hyman, Mark. *Food Fix: How to Save Our Health, Our Economy, Our Communities, and Our Planet—One Bite at a Time.* Little, Brown Spark, 2020.
    - This book offers solutions to improve health outcomes and create sustainable practices in food production and consumption.
- Hyman, Mark. *The Pegan Diet: 21 Practical Principles for Reclaiming Your Health in a Nutritionally Confusing World.* Little, Brown Spark, 2021.
    - Dr. Hyman presents a flexible and balanced approach to nutrition. The book includes practical tips and recipes to promote optimal health and longevity.
- Kern Lima, Jamie. *Worthy: Unlock Your Power to Change the World.* Hay House, 2024.
    - In this empowering memoir and guide, Jamie Kern Lima shares her personal struggles with self-worth and provides tools to help readers embrace their inherent value, break free from fear, and make meaningful contributions to the world.
- Leaf, Caroline. *Cleaning Up Your Mental Mess: 5 Simple, Scientifically Proven Steps to Reduce Anxiety, Stress, and Toxic Thinking.* Baker Books, 2021.
    - Dr. Leaf integrates neuroscience and practical tools to foster better mental health and overall well-being.
- Leaf, Caroline. *Think, Learn, Succeed: Understanding and Using Your Mind to Thrive at School, the Workplace, and Life.* Baker Books, 2018.
    - This book offers strategies for improving cognitive function and mental health to achieve personal and professional goals.

- Maté, Gabor. *When the Body Says No: Exploring the Stress-Disease Connection.*Wiley, 2003.
    - Dr. Gabor Maté delves into the relationship between stress and chronic illness, exploring how emotional and psychological stress can manifest in the body.
- Mylett, Ed. *The Power of One More: The Ultimate Guide to Happiness and Success*. Wiley, 2022.
    - Ed Mylett inspires readers to take control of their lives by embracing the concept of doing "one more" in various aspects of life.
- Neff, Kristin. *Self-Compassion: The Proven Power of Being Kind to Yourself.* HarperCollins, 2011.
    - Kristin Neff introduces the concept of self-compassion and how it can help you cope with chronic pain and emotional challenges.
- Nevin, Nancy. *Living with Chronic Pain: From OK to Despair and Finding My Way Back.* Beacon Books, 2018.
    - A heartfelt memoir and resource for those struggling with chronic pain.
- Ramey, Sarah. *The Lady's Handbook for Her Mysterious Illness.* Doubleday, 2020.
    - An illuminating and often humorous memoir about the challenges of living with an invisible illness.
- Shelton, Trent. *Protect Your Peace: How to Build Resilience and Calm in a Chaotic World*. Hay House, 2023.
    - Trent Shelton provides tools for setting boundaries and cultivating inner peace. His motivational advice is rooted in personal experiences.

- Van der Kolk, Bessel A. *The Body Keeps the Score: Brain, Mind, and Body in the Healing of Trauma.* Viking, 2014.
    - This book explores the relationship between trauma and the body, offering insights into the impacts of chronic pain and trauma on the brain.
- Winfrey, Oprah. *The Path Made Clear: Discovering Your Life's Direction and Purpose.* Flatiron Books, 2019.
    - A guide from Oprah Winfrey, helping readers navigate the journey of self-discovery and healing.

About the Author

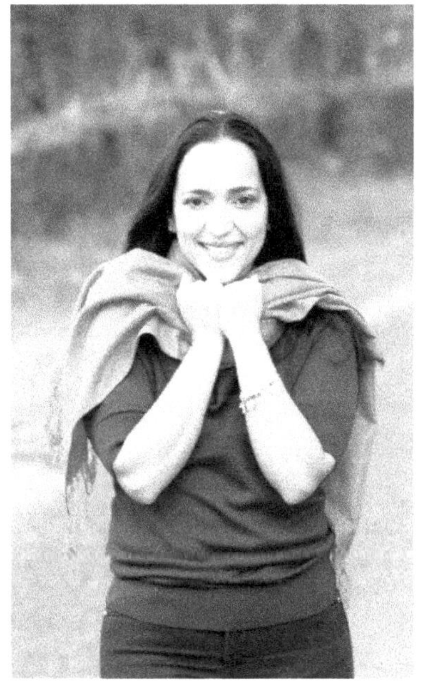

Michele Roys is an author, podcaster, and speaker with a passion for human connection. With a career spanning two decades across four continents, she has worked in human resources and leadership, helping people and organizations thrive. Her work in ten countries has given her a unique global perspective, which she now shares through her writing and speaking.

Beyond her corporate achievements, Michele co-founded *Hope in Motion*, a nonprofit organization in Ireland dedicated to empowering communities. Her commitment to service was recognized with the *University President Volunteer Award.* Though illness led her to step away from *Hope in Motion*, her dedication to helping others remains unwavering as she raises awareness for those living with chronic pain and invisible illness.

A graduate of the *University of Limerick*, Michele earned first-class honors in HR and Entrepreneurship and received multiple *Outstanding Scholar Awards* from the *Kemmy Business School*.

Michele lives in Limerick, Ireland, with her husband and two teenage sons.

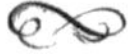

Connect with Michele:
Instagram: @michroys **Facebook:** michele.roys
YouTube: MicheleRoys **Podcast:** *The Michele Roys Show*

Michele is passionate about helping others rediscover joy, even in the midst of chronic pain. Through her book, podcast, and personal journey, she hopes to offer encouragement and practical support to those who need it most. To stay connected and receive a free set of affirmations for chronic pain warriors visit:
www.micheleroys.com